Pilates

for weight loss

Elise Watts

Published by Hinkler Books Pty Ltd
45–55 Fairchild Street
Heatherton Victoria 3202 Australia
www.hinkler.com.au

hinkler

Author: Elise Watts
Cover Design: Hinkler Design Studio
Designer: Sam Grimmer
Layout: Susanna Murray
Photography: Ned Meldrum
Prepress: Graphic Print Group
Clothing supplied by lululemon athletica

ISBN: 978 1 7418 3879 4

Printed and bound in China

Always do the warm up exercises before attempting any individual exercise. It is
recommended that you check with your doctor or health care professional before
commencing any exercise regime. While every care has been taken in the
preparation of this material, the publishers and their respective employees or
agents will not accept responsibility for injury or damage occasioned to any
person as a result of participation in the activities described in this book.

CONTENTS

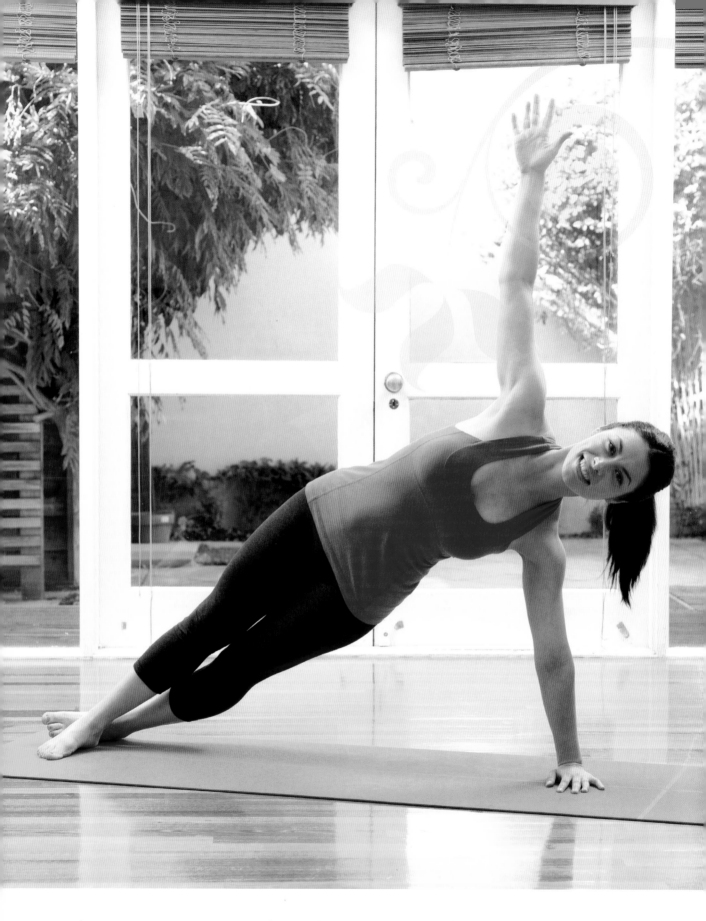

PILATES FOR WEIGHT LOSS

INTRODUCTION

Pilates is an outstanding method for creating perfect physical balance. For decades, performers, dancers and athletes have used the Pilates Method to transform their bodies by focusing on core strength and to enhance their wellbeing through the utilisation of breath and the controlled nature of the movements. Combined with a balanced diet and regular cardiovascular exercise, Pilates is an important contributor towards successful weight loss.

One of the reasons the Pilates Method is so successful is due to its origins. Its namesake and creator, Joseph Pilates, was influenced by many established exercise regimes such as martial arts, yoga and gymnastics. His initial concept for the method was to rehabilitate World War II soldiers, who needed to maximise their energy with the most effective results.

The method was enormously successful, proving that high intensity Pilates practice can literally transform the body in relatively few sessions. Joseph Pilates was often quoted as saying that as little as 30 hours of practice was all that was needed for a totally 'new body'. His personal method went on to lend itself superbly across many disciplines, and is especially known for its application to dance. Since his death in 1967, the Pilates Method has become so well known that it is practised worldwide, yet many people are still only just discovering the wonders that Pilates can produce for their mind and body.

Using a blend of traditional teachings and my own original practical applications, the program outlined in this book will help even the newest participant discover their body and its potential in a safe, enjoyable manner, with benefits that will be noticed immediately and can be sustained for the long term. Now you can utilise Pilates to lose weight, and to tone and create an efficient, healthy, strong physique!

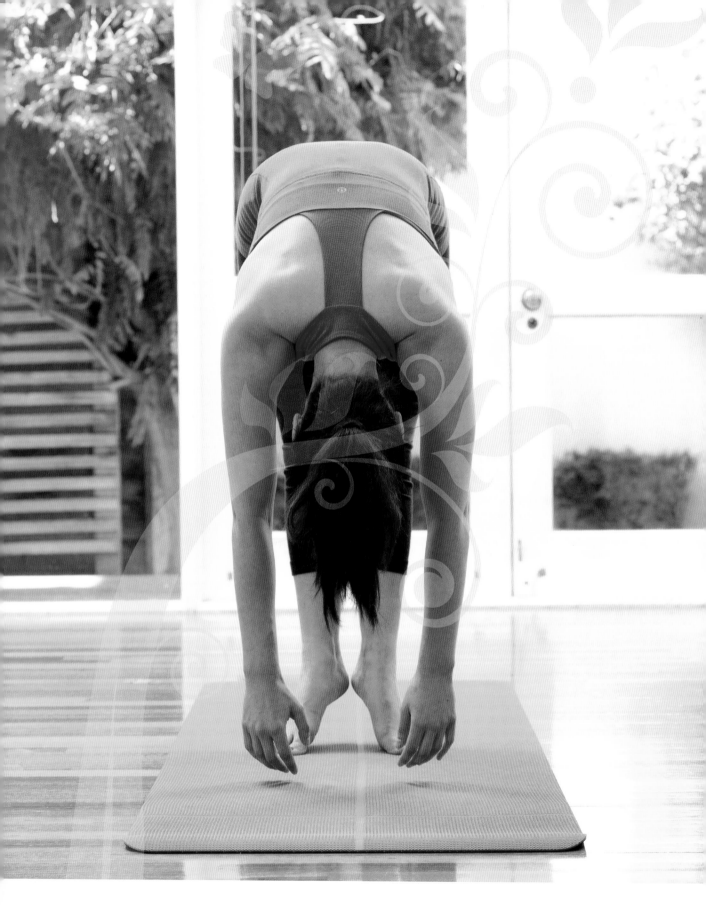

PILATES FOR WEIGHT LOSS

PILATES PRINCIPLES AND WEIGHT LOSS

CENTRING

Physical transformation begins with the deep internal pelvic, abdominal and gluteal muscle connections that provide the endurance necessary to sustain weight loss.

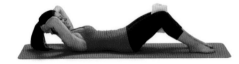

CONCENTRATION

The mind-body connection undoubtedly assists to transform the physical state, thinking your way towards a healthy, strong body through conscious, purposeful movement.

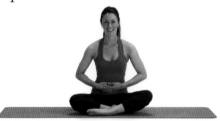

CONTROL

Deliberate placement and awareness of the body achieves the physical intelligence necessary for an efficient, lean physique.

PRECISION AND ALIGNMENT

Precision and alignment of all systems, from the skeletal and muscular to the digestive system, encourages the movement of lipids and caloric expenditure.

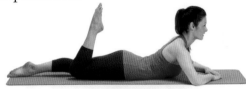

BREATHING

Proper breathing acts as a lymphatic and metabolic cleanser, establishing a clean, detoxified and healthy physical state.

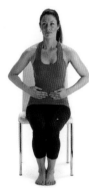

FLOW

Continuous, graceful and thoughtful movement utilises maximum energy, assisting weight loss through constant physical awareness.

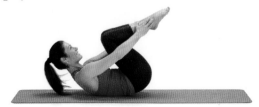

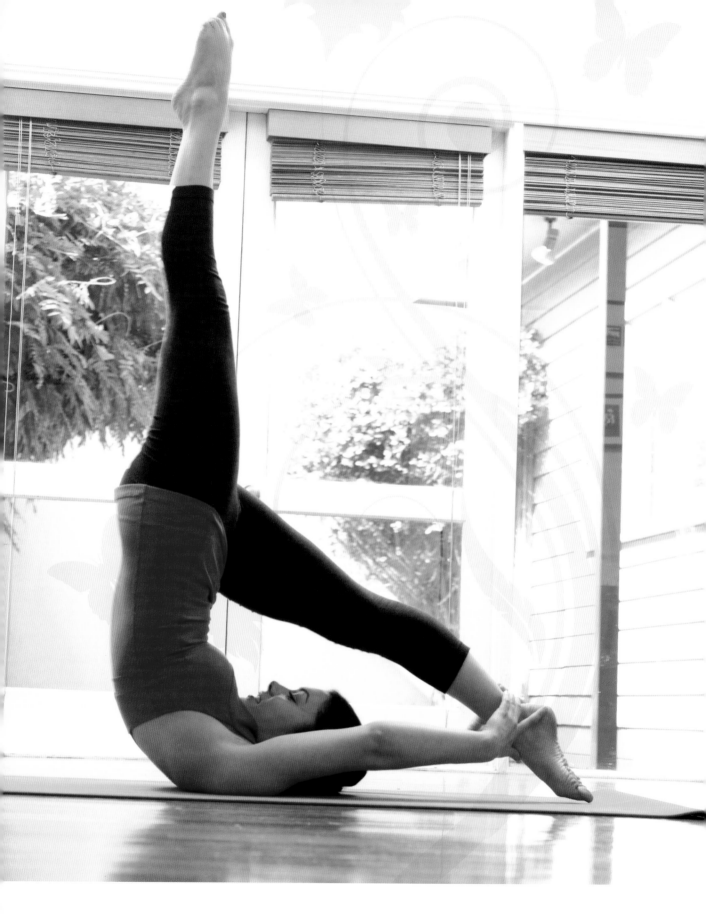

PILATES FOR WEIGHT LOSS

Integrated Weight Loss Approach

Along with consistent Pilates exercise, your weight-loss campaign should include:

- A healthy balanced diet
- Regular, safe cardiovascular exercise

Also consider incorporating any of the following exercises and activities into your weekly physical routine:

Traditional Cardio Exercise

Perform cardiovascular exercise, such as walking, running and skipping. If your fitness level allows, consider high-intensity short-duration interval training, known as fartlek training. This exercise style uses your stored energy as its main fuel source, leading to efficient shifting of excess weight.

Water Exercise

Swimming, water running and water aerobics: the water provides resistance and assists muscle toning, without impact, allowing safe, long-term practice, no matter what your fitness level.

Recreational Exercise

Dance classes, martial arts and team sports like netball, football and tennis make exercise fun and social, ensuring long-term application and sustained weight-loss results!

Use the Weight-Loss Planner at the end of this book to track your exercise routine. Safely building your way towards effective weight loss will ensure your results can be maintained for the long term.

Recovery

It is recommended that you practise Pilates no less than three times per week. At least one to two days per week should be devoted to recovery, allowing your body to process the physical changes taking place and to reserve your energy for your more active days. Spread your activities evenly throughout the week, listen to your body and rest when it tells you to so that you can stay fit and active for longer!

ESSENTIAL CONNECTIONS

Healthy, toned bodies are created from the inside out. The traditional Pilates Method utilises 'essential connections'. When practised throughout your workout, they establish clean muscle patterning, transforming your body through abdominal, gluteal and pelvic conditioning. It is recommended that the following connections be practised daily on commencement of your weight-loss program until they become automatic. They should also be executed as part of each exercise within the Pilates Method.

BREATH

Pilates breathing is defined by diaphragmatic and intercostal movement. It focuses on the lateral direction of the breath to release the thorax, open the airways and improve your posture. This relaxed breathing technique creates the focus and endurance to take your Pilates practice to an advanced level.

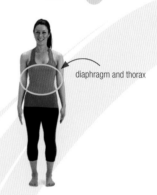

diaphragm and thorax

Pilates Breathing

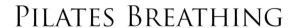

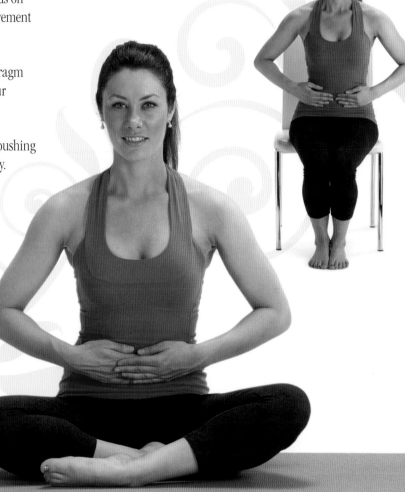

1 Seated cross-legged on the floor or on a chair, place your hands on your stomach and feel the movement of your diaphragm.

2 As you inhale, your diaphragm relaxes and drops into your lower belly.

3 As you exhale, it rises up, pushing the old air out of your body.

Tip

Allow your hands to fill up with your relaxed belly on the inhale. On the exhale, feel how the diaphragmatic movement draws the belly away.

Intensify

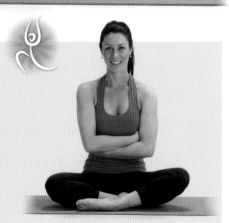

Cross your hands in front of your chest to feel the back and sides of your ribcage. As you inhale, try to expand the back of your ribs without the front of your ribs moving forward. This is known as 'lateral breathing'.

PELVIC FLOOR & GLUTEALS

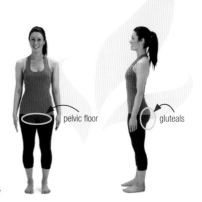
pelvic floor   gluteals

A large contributor to a flat, lean stomach is a strong, flexible pelvic floor. No matter how much abdominal work you do, without pelvic-floor awareness, your body cannot reach its physical potential. The following exercise flattens your stomach, stabilises the pelvis and spine, and also tones your inner thighs. You will need a solid chair to sit on and a rolled-up towel for this exercise.

SEATED PELVIC LIFT

1 Sitting on a chair, position your feet comfortably on the floor. Place a rolled-up towel between your knees and sit upright, with your spine elongated.

2 Become aware of the diamond-shaped bony landmarks at the base of your pelvis: the sitting bones, pubic bone and tailbone, where the pelvic floor muscles attach. This is often referred to as the 'pelvic diamond'.

3 Exhale, squeeze the towel gently and simultaneously lift your pelvic organs upwards, shrinking the pelvic diamond.

4 Inhale and gradually release, spreading your sitting bones and tailbone apart.

5 Repeat 10–12 times.

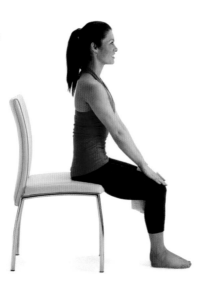

INTENSIFY

Gently engage the gluteal muscles that connect around the edge of your sitting bones as you exhale. This should be practised without contraction of your lumbar spine. It gives a sense of sitting up off the chair, and should not overstimulate the front of the thigh.

IMAGERY

Placing one hand on your lower stomach and the other on your lumbar spine, visualise your internal organs being vacuumed up your spine, as if travelling in a lift. By the end of your exhale, your organs should feel as though they've reached the top floor. Gradually lower your organs on your next inhale.

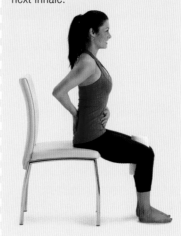

TIP

It is essential that you can clearly distinguish between the pelvic lift and the engagement of the lower gluteals. Practise of both muscle connections on their own is recommended.

Transversus Abdominis & Back Release

The transversus abdominis muscle acts as a postural stabiliser. It assists to narrow the waist, flatten the stomach and provide the strength for more advanced exercises. Historically, the transverse function in Pilates has simply been described as 'drawing the belly to the spine', but there is more to this connection than just the hollowing of your stomach. The following exercise focuses on the transversus abdominis with a lumbar fascia (the sheath that binds the muscles of the lower back together) release to create a dynamically intelligent spine.

transversus abdominis

Pelvic Funnel

1 Sitting on a chair or lying on your back, place a rolled-up towel between your knees. With your fingertips on your hipbones, check for alignment throughout the spine, and upper and lower limbs.

2 Exhale and lift your pelvic organs as practised in the Seated Pelvic Lift, this time encouraging your hipbones to slide apart. Aim for the back of the hipbones to slide apart and feel your sacrum and waistline widen.

3 Inhale and gently pull your hipbones towards each other again, while gradually releasing your pelvic floor. This should give the impression of your waistline narrowing.

4 Repeat 10 times.

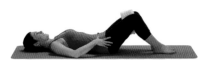

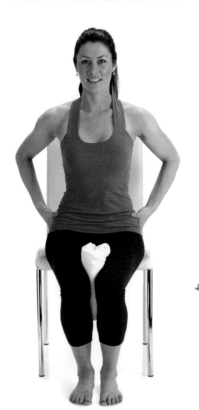

TIP
This movement may feel subtle, but its long-term effect is quite the opposite. If in doubt, visualise the movement to awaken the neuromuscular connections necessary.

INTENSIFY
Tilt your pelvis upwards as you exhale (pubic bone travelling to sternum and tailbone to back of knees) maintaining the lumbar–mat connection.

On the inhale, reverse this movement by sending your pelvis into an anterior tilt. As your pelvic floor is gradually released and your waist narrows, keep your lumbar region tension free as you gently press your tailbone into the floor. Your lumbar spine may come off the floor slightly.

IMAGERY
Your pelvis is a funnel: as the sitting bones open, the top of the funnel closes and vice versa.

HIP FLEXOR MOBILITY

Lengthening your hip flexors is one of the fastest ways to transform your thigh and pelvic region. Released hip flexors improve your Pilates technique and your overall physical performance. The following exercise is deceptively challenging. It requires coordination of muscle patterning, breath and balance to achieve abdominal control and pelvic stability. Practise this exercise daily until you can intensify the movement with ease.

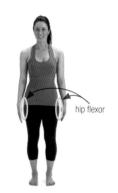

hip flexor

LEG FLOAT

1 Lying on your back with your legs bent and feet positioned on the floor hip-width apart, place your fingertips on the crease of your hips.

2 As you exhale, engage your stabilisers with your spine remaining long.

3 Fold one knee to your chest with your leg bent at a 90-degree angle.

4 Inhale to return to the starting position.

5 Repeat 10 times on each side.

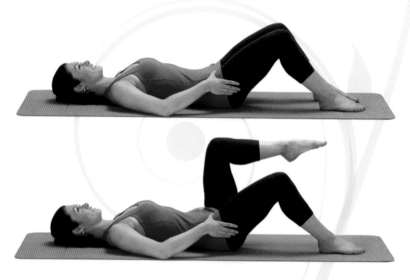

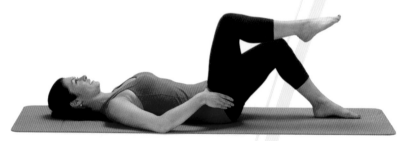

TIP
Ensure the front of your thighs relax throughout the movement to counter the tendency for your hip flexors to dominate by engaging your gluteals and hamstrings. Pelvic stability is achieved by maintaining pelvic floor connection throughout the exercise.

Simplify

Start from an assisted position, with your feet resting on a stack of pillows, books or a chair. This reduces the range of movement required to perfect the muscle patterning. Gradually reduce the height of the assisted position.

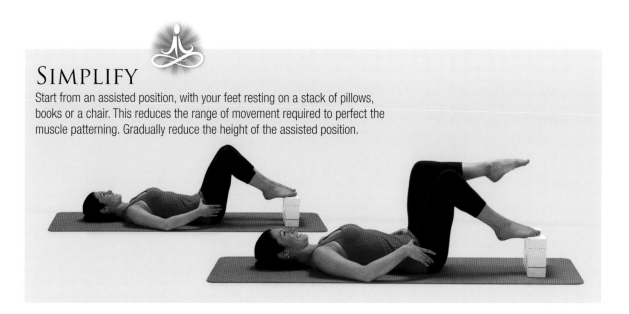

Intensify

Suspend one leg and bring your second leg into a leg float. Your belly must stay low throughout the movement, with your back relaxed and pelvic stability maintained on the exchange. Place your first leg down and then gently lower your second leg. Repeat on alternating sides.

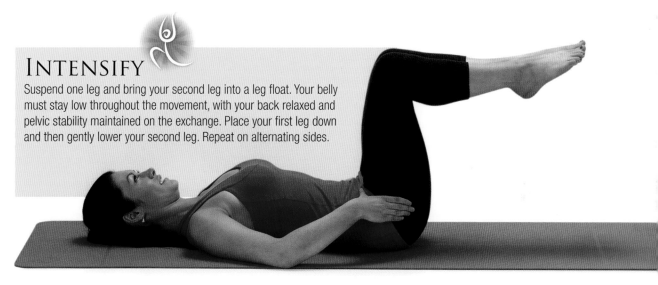

The gluteal, pelvic floor and transverse abdominal connections practised here should be performed with each exercise in this program. For simplicity's sake, these muscles will be referred to as the stabilisers throughout the rest of this program. Make a concerted effort to perform these multiple connections with each movement and each time you are instructed to engage your stabilisers.

Imagery

Visualise a marble balancing on your pubic bone. As you lift your leg, you roll the marble to your navel. The marble should stay in this position throughout the exercise, as your body appears completely still!

FUNDAMENTALS

The 'fundamentals' set up the basic structure for all the movements that follow in the Pilates weight-loss program. Take as long as you need to master these for the best results. When practised with conscious awareness of the essential connections, these exercises provide an intense toning workout.

CHEST LIFT

1 Lie on your back, with your legs bent and feet hip-width apart, a comfortable distance from your body.

2 Interlace your hands behind your head.

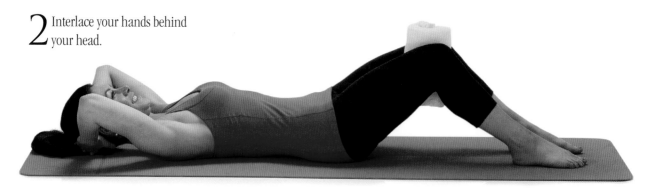

3 Exhale, engage your stabilisers and contract forward.

4 Inhale, hold and then exhale to return to the starting position, softening your lumbar spine into the floor.

5 Repeat 12–15 times.

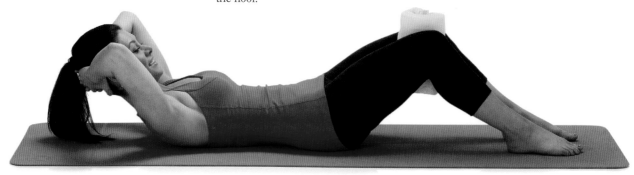

TIP

You can also perform this exercise with a rolled-up towel placed between your knees.

SIMPLIFY

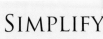

Lower on the inhale to reduce intensity.

INTENSIFY

Raise one or both legs to leg float position (90-degree bend), maintaining a lumbar release and increasing the connection to your stabilisers.

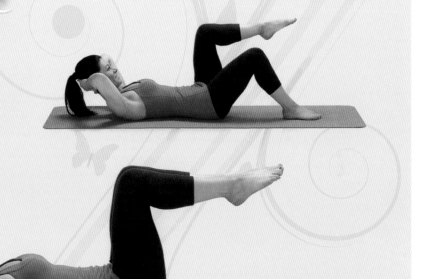

IMAGERY

Visualise a well in your stomach wall getting deeper as you curl up.

PELVIC CURL

1 Lie on your back with a neutral spine, with your legs bent and your heels a comfortable distance from your body. Relax your arms by your sides, with your palms open. Your back is long and your lumbar spine is relaxed.

2 Exhale and engage your stabilisers. Maintain this connection as you roll your tailbone towards the ceiling and peel your spine off the floor, one vertebra at a time. Your feet, upper back, neck and head should be all that remain on the floor.

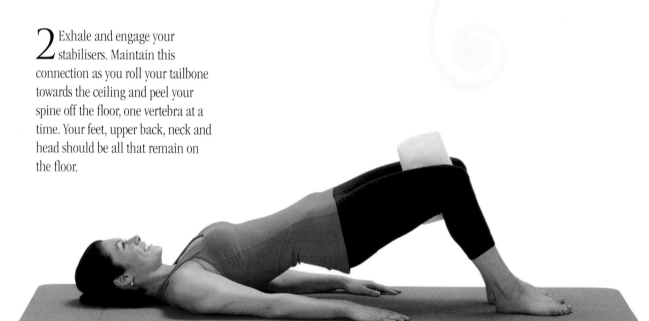

3 Hold this position at the top and inhale, checking that your lumbar spine is relaxed.

4 Exhale and roll down through each portion of your spine.

5 Return to the starting position on your next inhale.

6 Repeat 12–15 times.

TIP

Ensure lower limb alignment by placing a rolled-up towel between your knees. This encourages an adductor–pelvic floor connection, toning the inner thighs, glutes, hamstrings and stomach.

SIMPLIFY

Place your feet on a wall, with your legs in a 90-degree bend. You are less likely to engage your lumbar spine in this position.

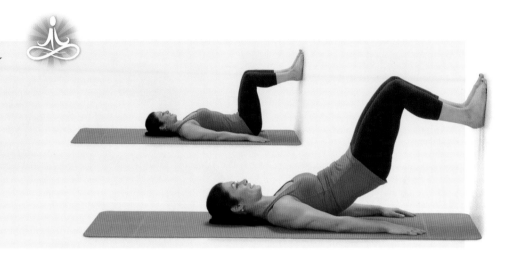

INTENSIFY

At the top of the movement, try a knee fold, maintaining pelvic stability and lumbar release.

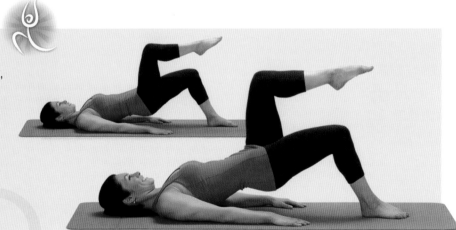

IMAGERY

Visualise your spine dangling from your pelvis at the top of the movement. This exercise should be felt in your glutes and hamstrings.

CAT STRETCH

1 Kneeling on all fours, place your wrists in line with your shoulders and your knees directly beneath your pelvis. Your spine should be flat and long. This is called the four-point kneeling position.

2 Exhale and engage your stabilisers and glutes, widening the hipbones as you flex your spine upward.

3 Inhale as you flatten your spine back to neutral, keeping your lumbar spine relaxed throughout.

4 Repeat 12–15 times, deepening the essential connection each time.

TIP
Aim for gluteal and hamstring activity throughout.

SIMPLIFY
Begin by practising the Pelvic Funnel as described earlier in Essential Connections on all fours, before adding the flexion of your lumbar spine.

IMAGERY
Visualise your navel being magnetically drawn to the ceiling, releasing your lumbar spine further on the exhale.

INTENSIFY
On the inhale, gradually release your sitting bones and draw your hipbones together, bringing your spine into an extension.

Spine Twist

1 Lie on your back with your arms extended diagonally at each side and your palms facing down. Position your feet and knees together, with your knees bent at right angles.

2 Inhale and sequentially roll your spine to one side, keeping your knees aligned and your shoulders on the floor at all times. Ensure that when rolling across, you move your knees and feet first, followed by your hips, waist and finally ribcage.

3 Exhale and roll sequentially back through the spine to the starting position. When rolling back, move your ribcage first, then your waist, hips and lastly your knees and feet.

4 Repeat 12–15 times, alternating sides.

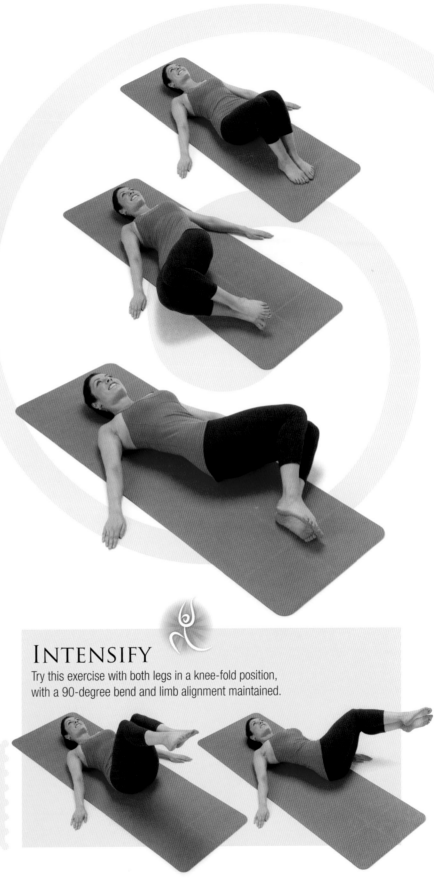

Tip
Use a flexed lumbar spine to imprint your back from your thorax to pelvis, section by section.

Imagery
Feel your vertebrae rotate like a necklace of cotton spools, rolling them across from top to bottom and back again.

Intensify
Try this exercise with both legs in a knee-fold position, with a 90-degree bend and limb alignment maintained.

Lateral Leg Float

1 Lie on your side, with your underneath arm extended away from your body and your head resting on top of it.

2 Use your top arm to support your body with your fingertips positioned on the floor in front of your navel.

3 Place your feet in a 'V' position with your heels together, top leg toes facing the ceiling and lower leg toes facing the floor.

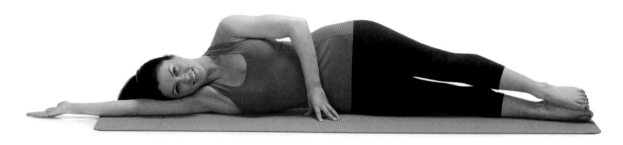

4 Exhale and connect to your core stabilisers as you raise your top leg to just above hip height, rotating the knee and big toe towards the ceiling and deeply activating your hip rotators and glutes.

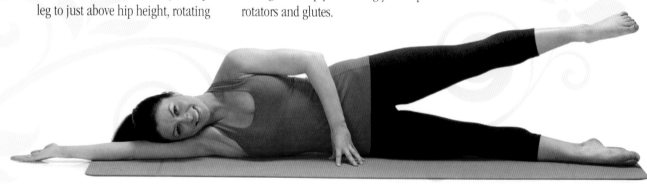

5 Inhale to lower to the starting position.

6 Maintain pelvic stability throughout this movement. While you raise your top leg, your pelvis should remain aligned in its starting position, with your lumbar spine rested.

7 Repeat 12 times on both sides.

TIP

Connect to the underneath oblique muscles of your abdomen prior to moving your top leg.

SIMPLIFY

Position your body against a wall for greater alignment feedback and balance.

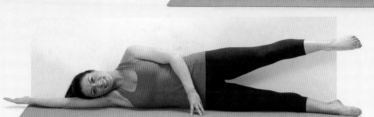

INTENSIFY

Raise your support arm to your hip or towards the ceiling for an extra balance challenge.

IMAGERY

Visualise your body from all directions. Allow your body to elongate as the movement takes place.

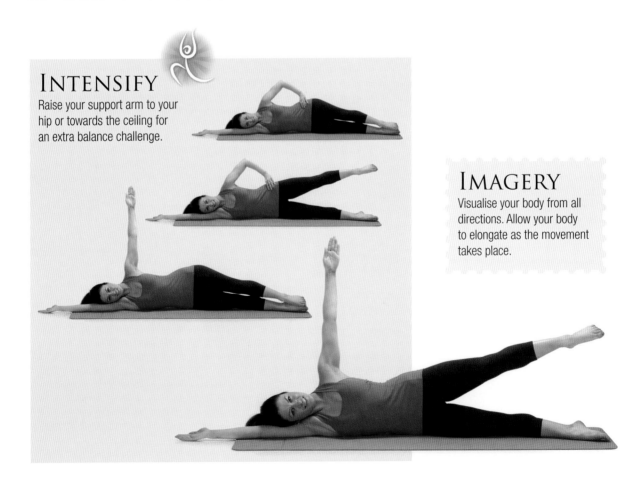

INTERMEDIATE CHALLENGE

Now that you have mastered some basic Pilates exercises, you are ready to create intensity with the use of lever changes and variations.

CHEST LIFT WITH LEG FLOAT

1 Lie on your back with your left hand behind your head and your right hand on the edge of your sitting bone. Bend both legs, with feet relaxed and placed a comfortable distance from your body.

2 Exhale and contract forward, engaging your stabilisers and lifting your head and chest off the floor.

3 Simultaneously fold your right knee as your fingers monitor your gluteal function, which should remain prominent throughout.

4 Inhale to lower your leg to the starting position.

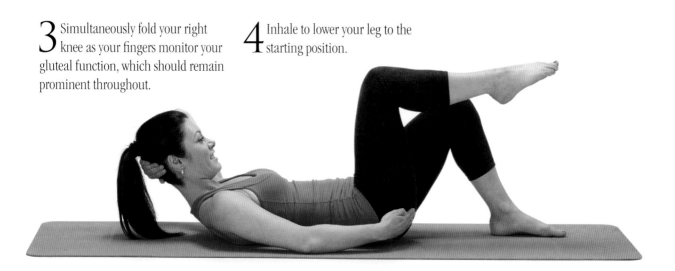

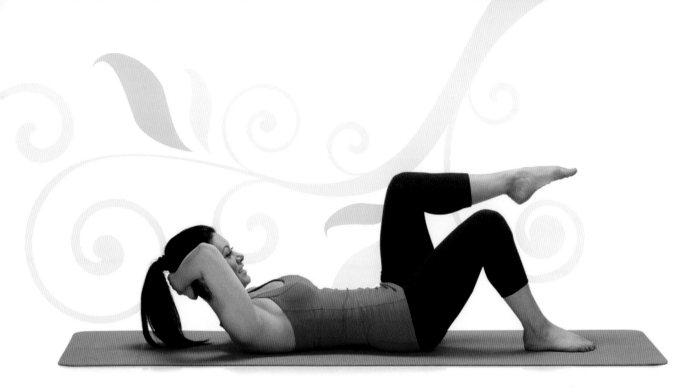

5 Repeat 8 times on your right leg before reversing the movement for another 8 repetitions. With the right leg held in the raised position, the leg lowers as you exhale, and contracts and rises as you inhale and your head and chest return to the starting position.

6 Repeat this exercise with the left leg 8 times in each direction.

INTENSIFY

After floating your knee off the floor, extend your leg and lower it to the floor while maintaining a chest lift. This exercise requires a longer exhale and will load your abdomen much more, so strong core stabilisation, glute and pelvic floor activation is required to keep your back long and relaxed.

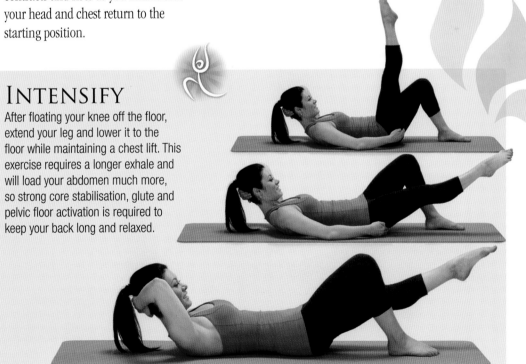

Roll Backs with Hamstring Stretch

1 Sitting across a mat, place your hands on your thighs. Keep your feet flat on the ground, directly below your knees, and your spine long. Your knees and feet are together.

2 Exhale, engage your stabilisers and widen your hipbones as you roll back, tucking your tail under.

3 Inhale and hold this position as you flex your feet.

4 Exhale to extend your legs and curl forward, maintaining flexed feet and enjoying a hamstring stretch.

5 Inhale to return to the starting position.

6 Repeat 12 times.

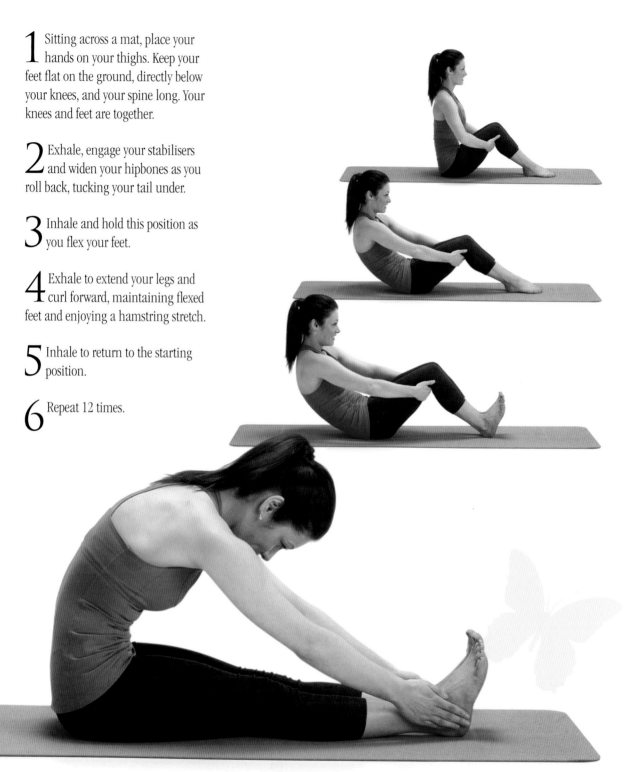

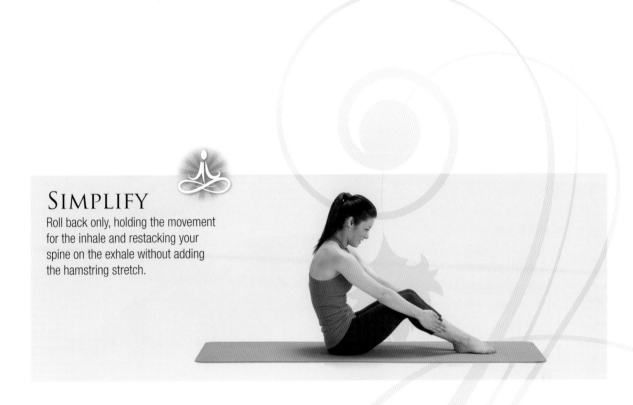

SIMPLIFY

Roll back only, holding the movement for the inhale and restacking your spine on the exhale without adding the hamstring stretch.

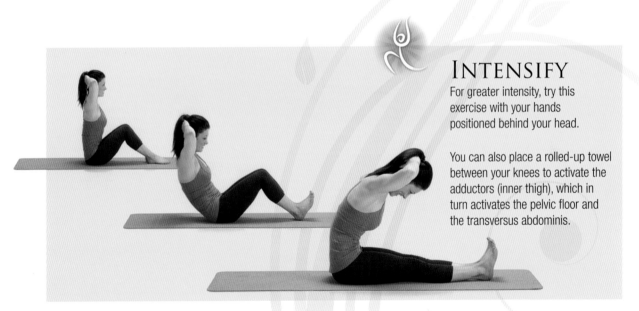

INTENSIFY

For greater intensity, try this exercise with your hands positioned behind your head.

You can also place a rolled-up towel between your knees to activate the adductors (inner thigh), which in turn activates the pelvic floor and the transversus abdominis.

IMAGERY

As you tuck your tail under, visualise your spine making a crescent-moon shape, deepening into your flexion as you stretch forward.

Long Clam

1 Lie on your side, with your knees stacked and your heels in line with your sitting bones.

2 Exhale and open your top knee high towards the ceiling. Do not shift or move the pelvis.

3 Inhale as your thigh remains in this position and extend your leg, activating your deep hip rotators and glutes.

4 Exhale, bending and returning your leg back to the Clam position.

5 Inhale and return your leg to the starting position.

6 Repeat 12–15 times.

Simplify
Omit the leg extension.

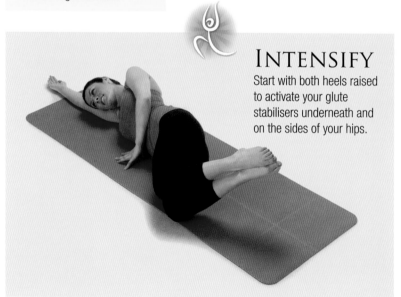

Intensify
Start with both heels raised to activate your glute stabilisers underneath and on the sides of your hips.

Imagery
Visualise your muscles wrapping around your femur bone like curling ribbon, spiralling your knee to the ceiling.

SINGLE LEG KICK

1 Lie on your stomach. Place your hands slightly in front of your body, angling them inwards. Rest your head on your hands, with your knees and ankles together.

2 Inhale as you lift your breastbone and extend your spine to half Cobra, pressing your hands and elbows into the ground. Lift only as high as you can with your back remaining tension free.

3 As you exhale, bend your right knee three times, keeping your foot slightly pointed but relaxed. Maintain the alignment of your leg as you pulse your breath for three counts during this leg movement.

4 Inhale as you lower your leg and extend your spine slightly higher.

5 Exhale and return to the starting position, preparing to repeat with your left leg.

6 Repeat both movements 8 times on each leg, alternating legs as you go.

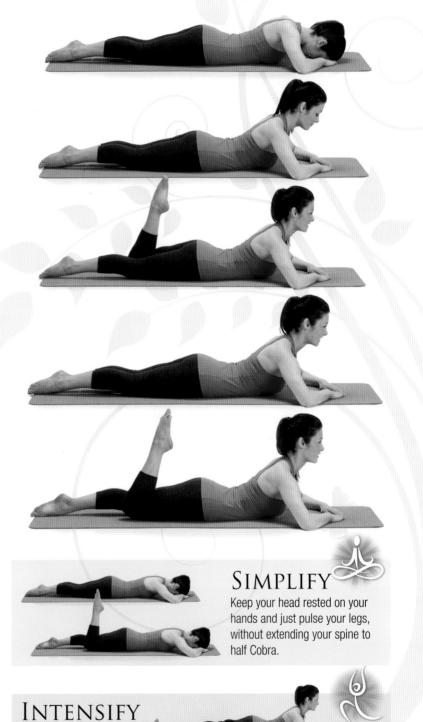

SIMPLIFY
Keep your head rested on your hands and just pulse your legs, without extending your spine to half Cobra.

TIP
Minor flexion of the lumbar spine assists comfort and reduces lumbar back tension.

INTENSIFY
Maintain lifted chest throughout the exercise.

Cat Stretch Push Up

1 Begin in the four-point kneeling position. Kneeling on all fours, place your wrists in line with your shoulders and your knees directly beneath your pelvis. Your spine is flat and long.

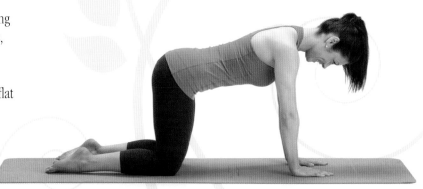

2 Exhale and round your lumbar spine, initiating movement from your glutes and pelvic floor.

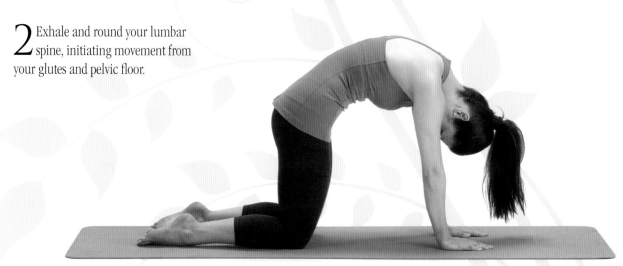

3 Maintain this gluteal connection as you slowly sit back on your heels into a resting pose.

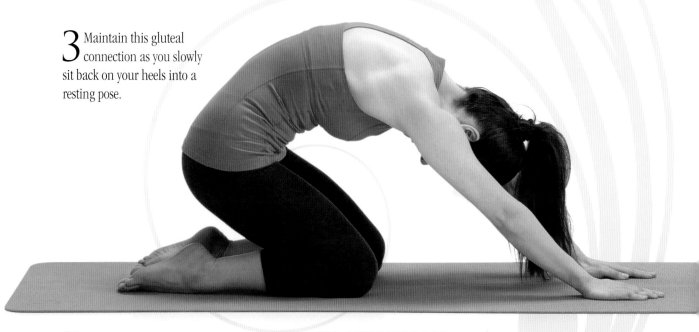

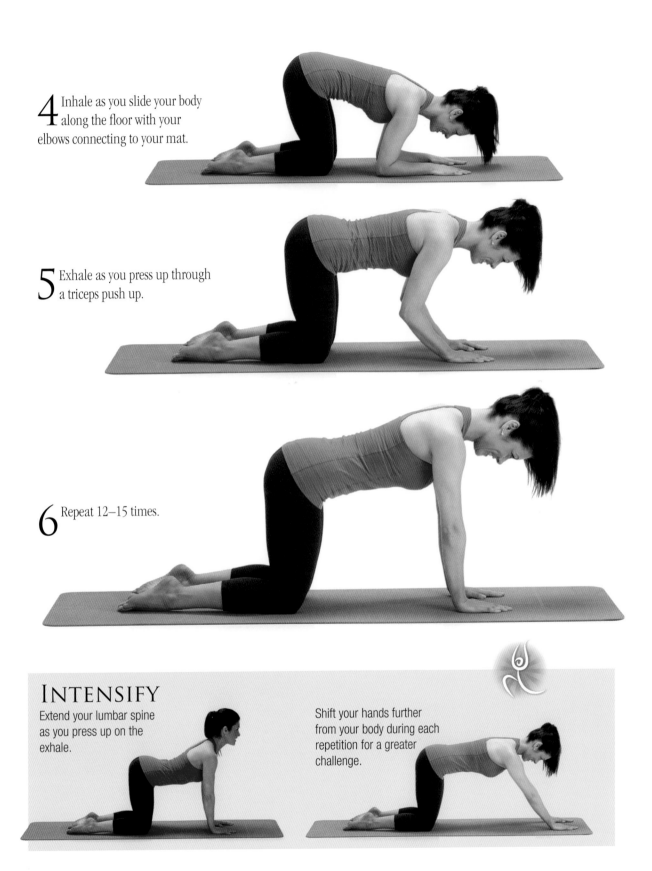

4 Inhale as you slide your body along the floor with your elbows connecting to your mat.

5 Exhale as you press up through a triceps push up.

6 Repeat 12–15 times.

INTENSIFY

Extend your lumbar spine as you press up on the exhale.

Shift your hands further from your body during each repetition for a greater challenge.

COBRA

1 Lying prone, place your hands slightly in front of your body, angled inwards, with your legs hip-width apart.

2 Inhale, lift your breastbone and extend your spine, pressing your hands and elbows into the ground. Your shoulders should slide down your back as you inhale, working the thoracic spine. Lift your breastbone only as high as you can with your back remaining tension free.

3 Avoid lumbar tension by releasing your sitting bones and gently engaging your abdominals.

4 Exhale and lower to the starting position. Repeat 12–15 times.

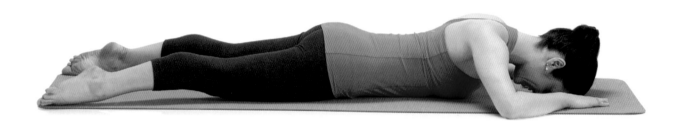

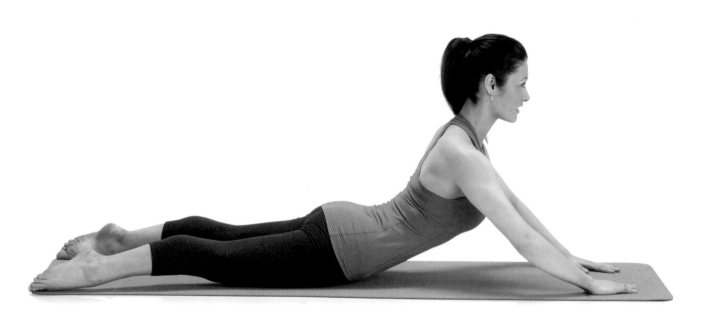

TIP

Working less from the muscles and more from the bones will produce greater results.

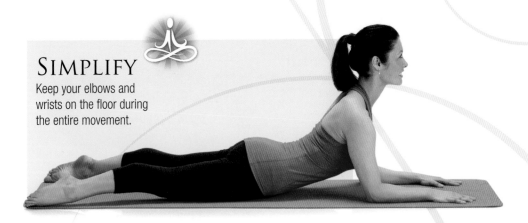

SIMPLIFY

Keep your elbows and wrists on the floor during the entire movement.

INTENSIFY

Gradually work to extend your arms completely, while ensuring your lumbar spine remains soft.

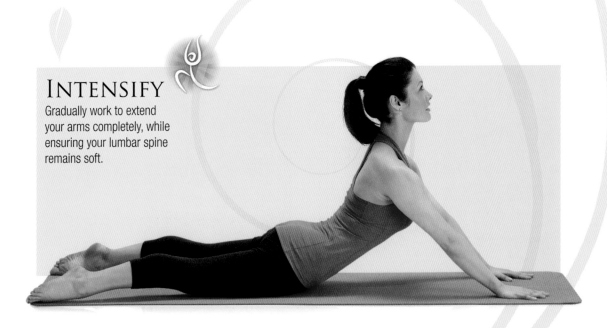

PRONE EXTENSION WITH ARM LIFT

1 Lie prone on your stomach with your arms extended along your sides. Position your legs hip-width apart with your heels facing each other.

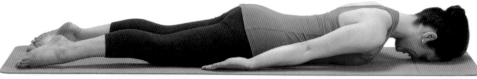

2 Inhale, gently connecting your abdominals and allowing your gaze to travel upwards as you elevate your upper spine and head off the floor.

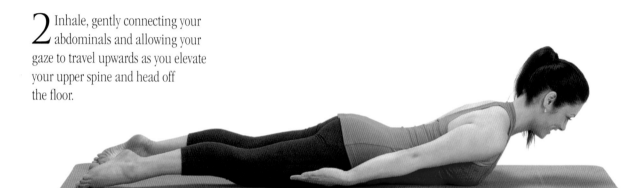

3 As you rise, simultaneously lift and reach your arms towards your toes. Your shoulder blades should remain separated and flat upon your ribcage.

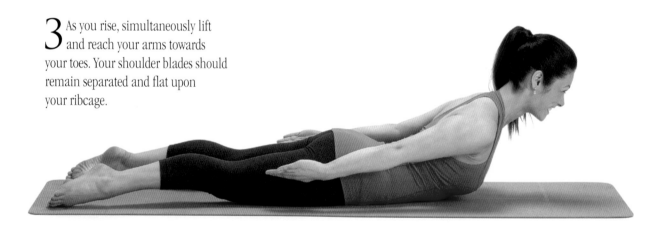

4 Exhale and lower with control to the starting position.

5 Repeat 12 times.

TIP

As you rise, slide your shoulder blades down your spine and outwards, engaging your lats and serratus muscles (which run along the sides of the back from the shoulder blades to the lower back).

SIMPLIFY

Open your legs wider than hip width and reduce the height of the movement.

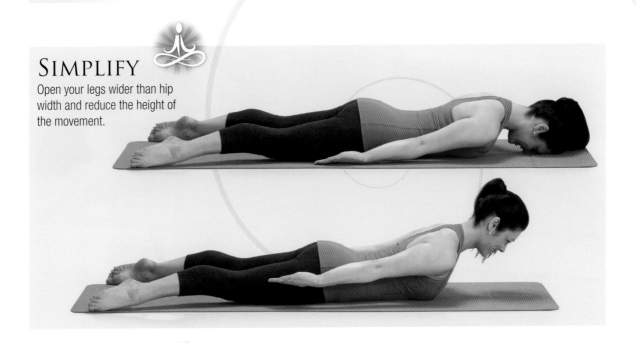

INTENSIFY

Hold each repetition at the top for an inhale and exhale before you lower to the floor. Use the extra breath to observe any unnecessary tension in your back.

IMAGERY

Rely on the bones and relax the muscles to create greater muscle fatigue through your upper back.

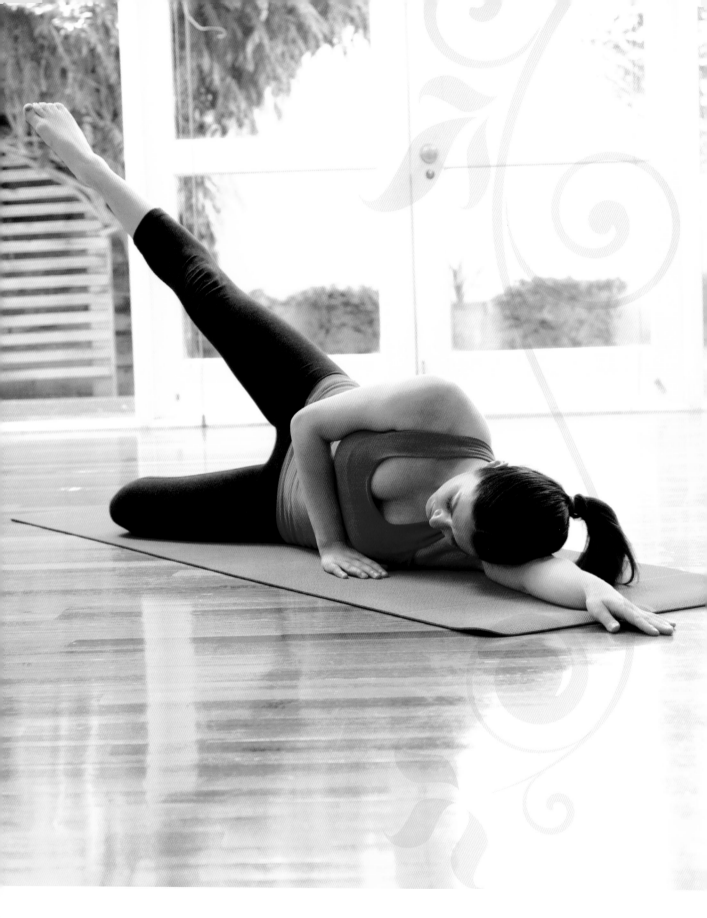

Dynamic Challenge

Tip

Press your legs into your hands, and with equal strength use your arms to pull your legs towards you. This constant push-pull creates an excellent abdominal connection and overall body toning.

The exercises in this series are defined by their functionality and flow. Control and strength are required to make them appear effortless.

Rolling

1 In a seated position, draw your knees close to your chest, with your ankles and knees together. Place your hands around your ankles, engaging your stabilisers throughout this exercise.

2 Inhale as you roll backwards along your spine to the edge of your shoulder blades.

3 Exhale to roll and balance on your sitting bones with your feet positioned just off the floor.

4 Repeat 12–15 times.

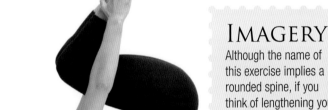

Imagery

Although the name of this exercise implies a rounded spine, if you think of lengthening your spine, this movement will be more streamlined.

Simplify

Place your hands higher on your shins.

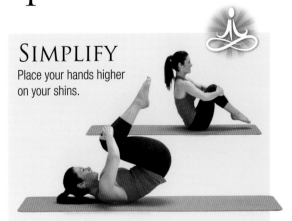

Intensify

Cross your hands in front of your ankles.

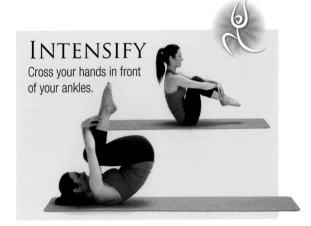

LATERAL ADDUCTOR LIFT

1 Lie on your side, with your bottom arm extended away from your body and your head resting on top of it. Position your legs slightly in front of your body line. Use your top arm to support your body, with your fingertips positioned on the floor in front of your navel.

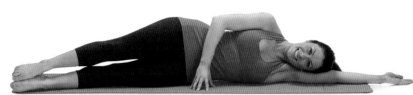

2 Engage your stabilisers and raise your top leg; this leg will remain here throughout the exercise.

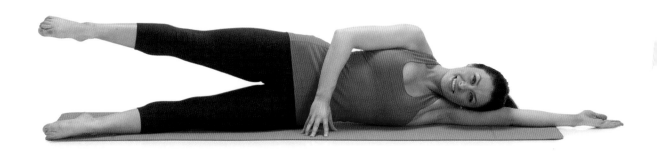

3 Exhale, engaging your stabilisers again as you lift your bottom leg to meet your top leg. Keep your lumbar spine soft as you extend both legs away from you.

4 Inhale and lower just your bottom leg.

5 Repeat 12–15 times on both sides.

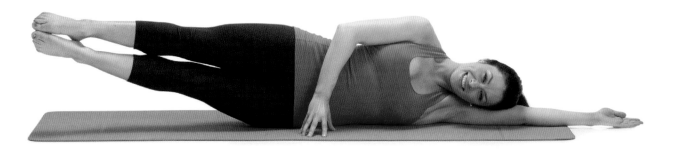

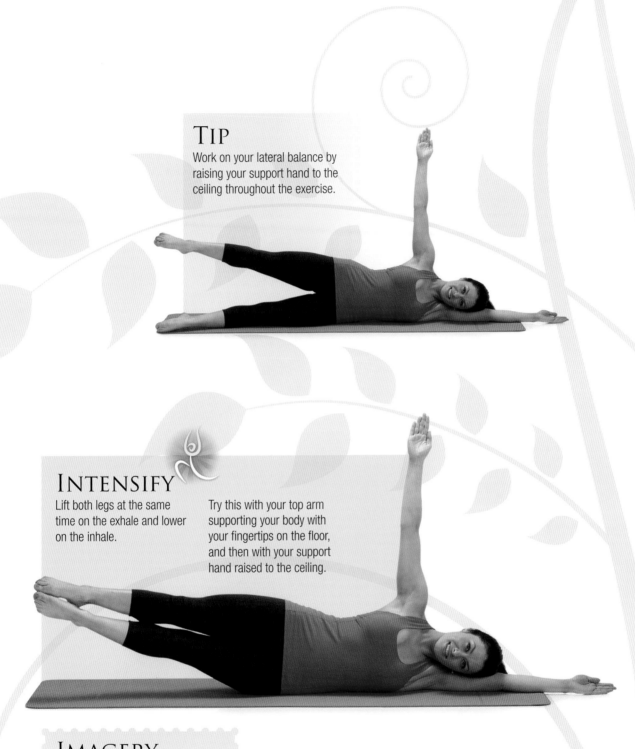

TIP

Work on your lateral balance by raising your support hand to the ceiling throughout the exercise.

INTENSIFY

Lift both legs at the same time on the exhale and lower on the inhale.

Try this with your top arm supporting your body with your fingertips on the floor, and then with your support hand raised to the ceiling.

IMAGERY

During each repetition, visualise your body as a piece of elastic being stretched longer from head to toe.

SIDE BICYCLE

If you have experienced prior knee injuries, you should reduce the range of movement described in the following exercise or omit it due to deep knee flexion. This movement should not aggravate the knee joint.

1 Lie on your side with your bottom arm extended away from your body and your head resting on top of your extended arm. Position your lower leg so that it is bent at a right angle to your hip, with your top leg extended away from your body. Use your top arm to support your body, with your fingertips positioned on the floor in front of your navel.

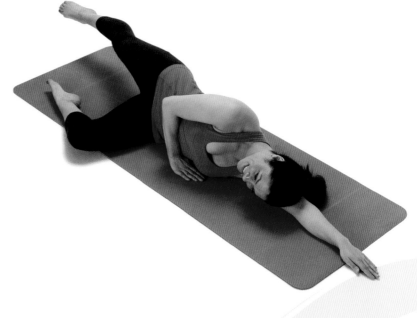

2 Keeping your top leg long, move into a hip extension as you exhale and bring your leg behind the line of your body as far as you can without shortening your lumbar spine.

3 With your glutes and hamstrings active, flex your foot. Without changing the position of your thigh, draw your heel to your bottom, activating a quadriceps stretch.

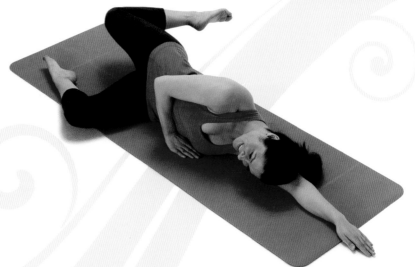

4 Keep your heel as close to your bottom as possible as you draw the knee towards your chest. Extend the leg to the front of your body and point your toes, beginning the cycle again by pushing the leg through the air until the leg passes the body line.

5 Repeat the exercise 16 times in total on each leg; 8 times forward and 8 times in the reversed direction. Your hips should remain aligned throughout.

IMAGERY
Visualise your lower body underwater, with your leg pushing against the force of the water.

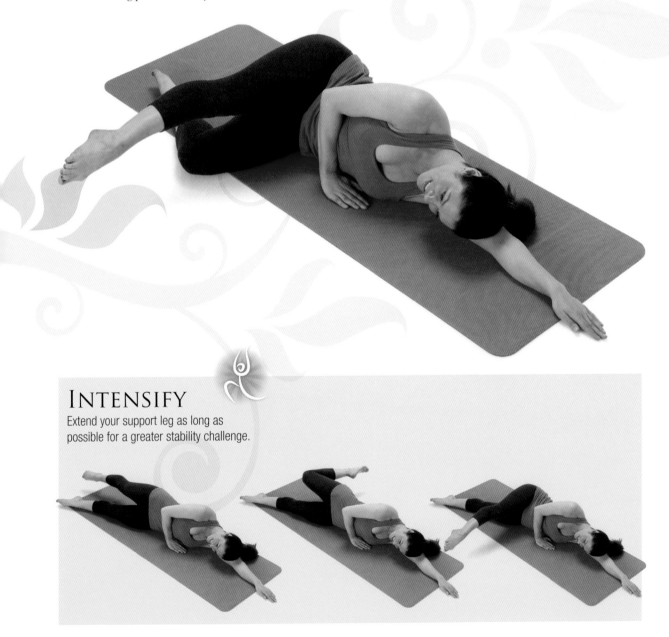

INTENSIFY
Extend your support leg as long as possible for a greater stability challenge.

SWAN

If you have experienced disc injury, take care in this next exercise. Simplify where necessary and support your spine with your stabilisers.

1 Lie on your stomach, with your arms extended in front of you and your legs wide and turned out.

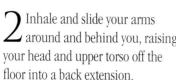

2 Inhale and slide your arms around and behind you, raising your head and upper torso off the floor into a back extension.

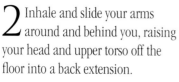

3 Raise one leg as you sustain the back extension.

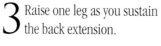

4 Exhale and raise the other leg, still sustaining the back extension.

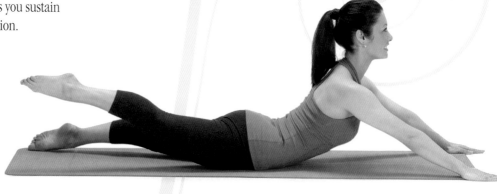

5 Inhale to lower your first leg.

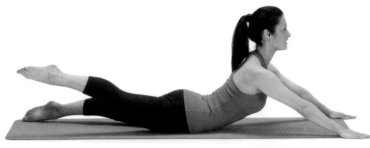

6 Exhale and lower your second leg and return to the starting position.

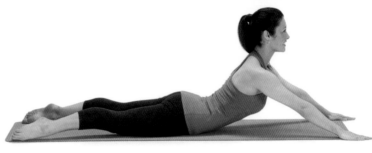

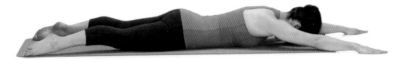

7 Repeat this exercise 8–10 times, alternating your starting leg, then try raising and lowering both legs simultaneously for 8–10 repetitions.

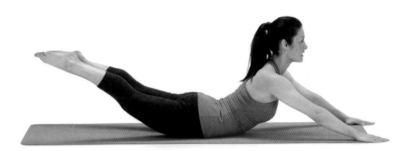

SIMPLIFY

Keep your upper torso on the floor, with your forehead resting on your hands, and just focus on your glutes and the leg raises.

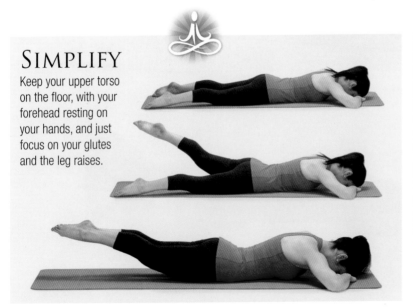

INTENSIFY

At the end of the repetitions, add some heel beats: 20–30 quick movements, drawing together the heels, with your upper body low to the floor.

TIP

Length is more important than height in this exercise.

Stabiliser Challenge

The exercises in this series promote postural stabiliser strength and create great overall toning effects.

Front Support Walks

1 Start in the four-point kneeling position. Lower your upper body onto your elbows and slide your knees out from under your hip line so your spine is flat.

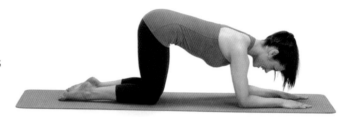

2 Tucking your toes under for grip, extend one leg straight so your entire body makes a diagonal line from heel to head.

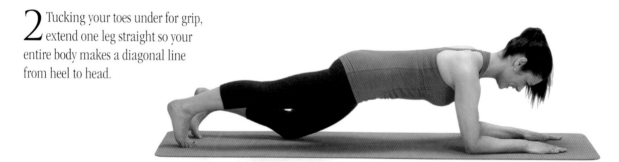

3 Exhale, engage your stabilisers and straighten the other leg.

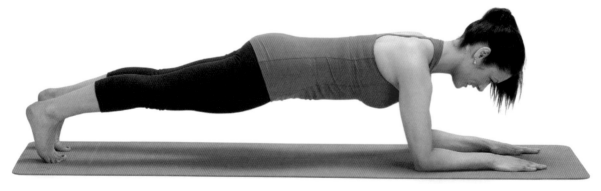

4 Inhale and lower the first leg. Exhale and lower the second leg. Inhale, extend the alternate leg out and repeat the walks in reverse.

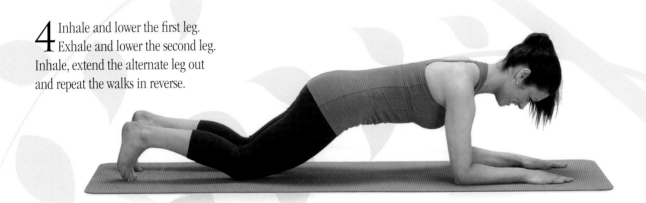

5 Repeat the walks a total of 5 times, alternating the starting leg each time.

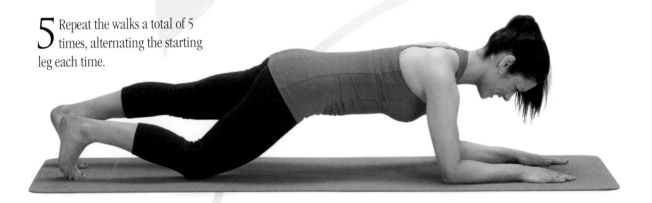

TIP

The spine should not reveal any change taking place. Use your pelvic and abdominal connections to make the exercise as seamless as possible.

INTENSIFY

Omit the walks and maintain front support.

Try the walks with straight arms.

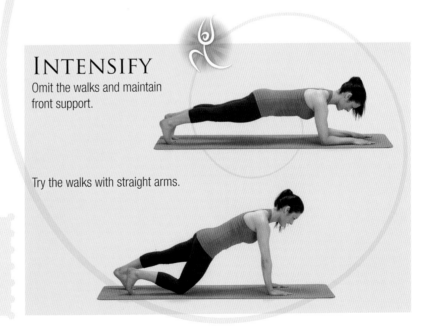

IMAGERY

Imagine that you are balancing a crystal ball on your spine, trying not to let it roll off!

SIDE SUPPORT

1 Sitting on your side, stack your knees and align your heels with your sitting bones. Your support arm should be straight, with your wrist directly underneath your shoulder. Rest your other arm on your ankle.

2 Exhale, engage your stabilisers and raise your hips to the ceiling, reaching your non-supporting arm over your head. Your shoulder should simultaneously slide down your back to support your body.

3 Inhale to maintain and increase the lateral stretch.

4 Exhale to lower and inhale to prepare to repeat the exercise.

5 Repeat this exercise a total of 12 times on each side.

TIP

Keep your hips and shoulders aligned from top and bottom to ensure ultimate balance.

SIMPLIFY

Try resting on your elbow to reduce the load.

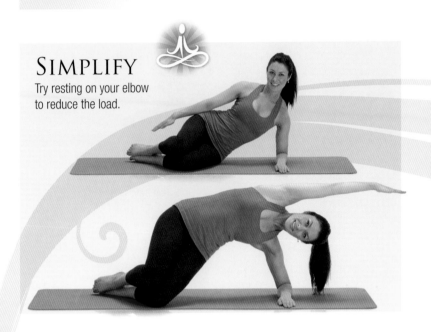

INTENSIFY

Lie on your side and place your lower arm long along the floor under your head. Rest your head on your outstretched arm and place your other arm in front of your body, palm down on the floor.

Exhale and slide your lower arm towards you along the floor as you raise your torso up into a very challenging side stretch. Keep the palm of your other hand on the floor. Inhale to lower with control.

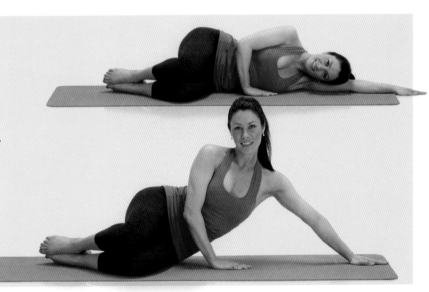

IMAGERY

Visualise your body in a thin corridor. Avoid hitting the sides by staying directly in the middle.

HINGE PRESS

If you have experienced prior knee injuries, you should omit this exercise due to its deep knee flexion. This movement should not aggravate the knee joint.

1 Begin by kneeling and then sit back on your heels with your arms resting by your sides.

2 Exhale, engage your stabilisers and tuck your tail under, lengthening your lumbar spine. Raise your arms to shoulder height, keeping your shoulders and neck relaxed as you simultaneously rise up to a kneeling position.

3 Inhale to open your sitting bones as you slightly extend your spine and return to sit back on your heels.

4 Repeat 12 times.

TIP

To maximise the effectiveness of this glute exercise, ensure your glute muscles are firing prior to movement and initiate the press with a gradual rise of your pelvic floor.

SIMPLIFY

Omit the arm movements and use a mirror to correct your alignment.

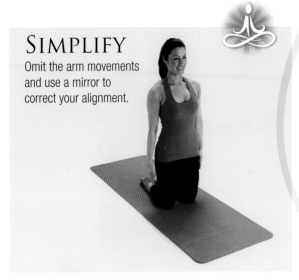

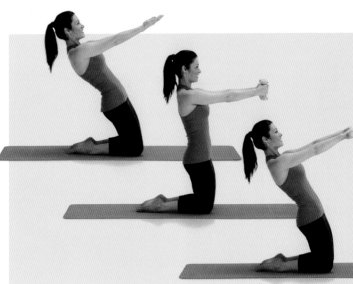

INTENSIFY

Lower yourself into an increased hinge position so that your body leans on a diagonal line from your knees. Maintaining this pose throughout the exercises will challenge your quadriceps, gluteals and spine stabilisers, and also increases the work through your chest and arms.

Use light hand weights (0.5–2kg) when raising your arms.

IMAGERY

Visualise your spine getting longer like a piece of elastic when you rise up to kneel.

ARMS IN HINGE

Maintaining the previously described hinge press position, try 8–10 repetitions of the following arm exercises, lowering from the hinge and sitting back on your heels at each change of exercise.

1 **Chest Opening:** Inhale and open your arms to a 'T' position. Exhale to draw your arms back to centre.

2 **Arm Float:** Inhale to float your arms to the ceiling. Exhale to lower your arms down by your hips.

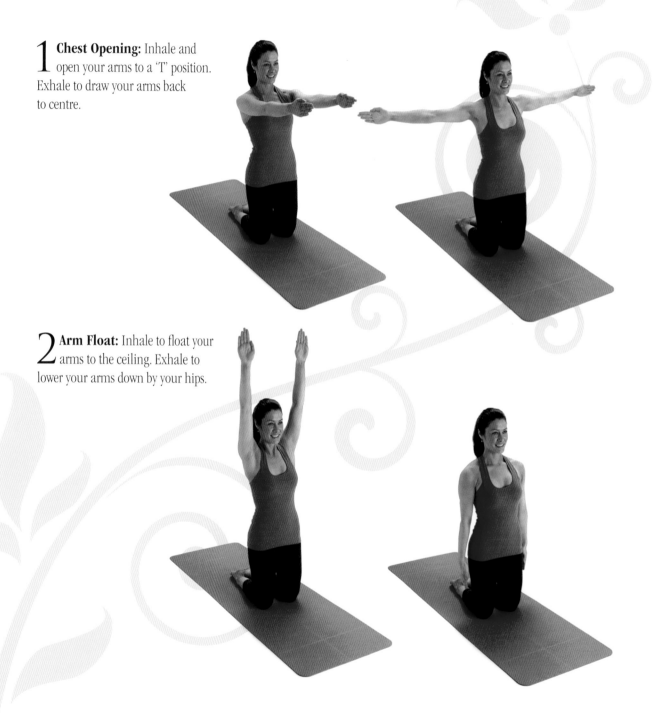

3 Rotator Cuff: Inhale to open your arms to the side, with your palms facing up and your elbows tucked in. Exhale to draw your arms back to your sides with your palms facing up.

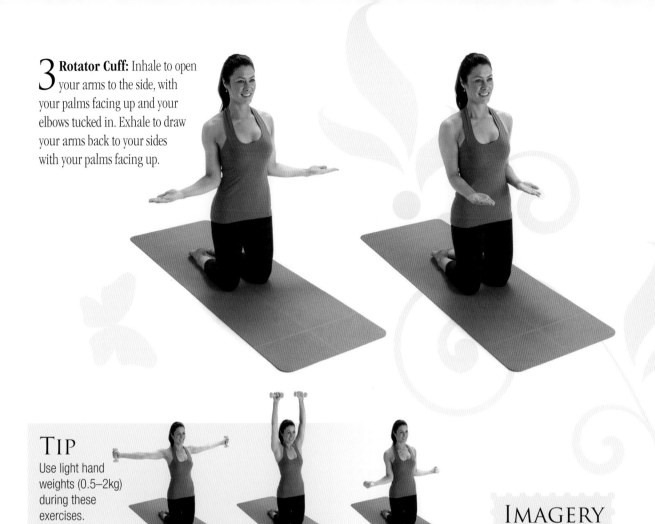

TIP
Use light hand weights (0.5–2kg) during these exercises.

IMAGERY
Visualise your body as very light, floating like a feather towards the sky.

INTENSIFY
Lower yourself into an increased hinge position so that your body leans on a diagonal line from your knees.

Add light hand weights as you lean on the diagonal to further increase the intensity.

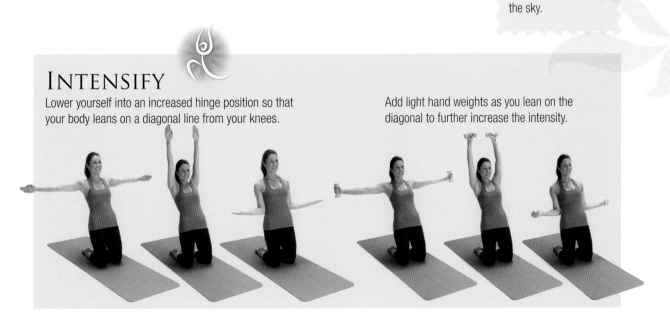

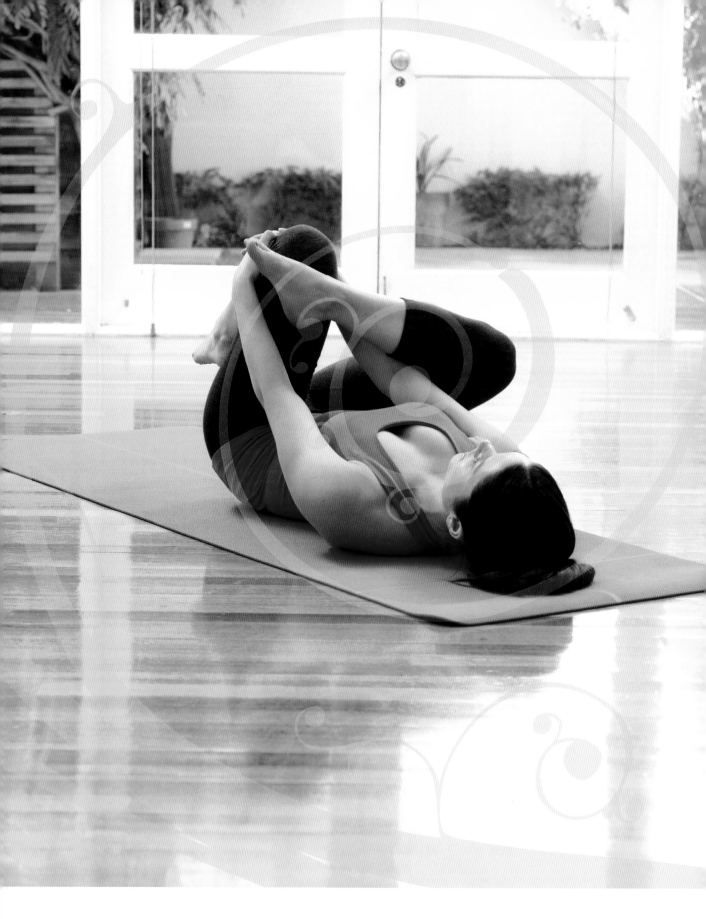

PILATES FOR WEIGHT LOSS

COOL DOWN

Stretching is an important component to any physical program, as it allows the larger external muscles to release and lengthen, creating a longer, leaner look. It also restores the body, making it ready for your next workout.

GLUTEAL STRETCH

1 Lying on your back, cross one leg in front of the other and reach for your ankles or toes, drawing both feet towards your body.

2 Maintain this stretch for 1–2 minutes.

3 Repeat on the other leg.

TIP
Use your breath to relax deeper into the stretch.

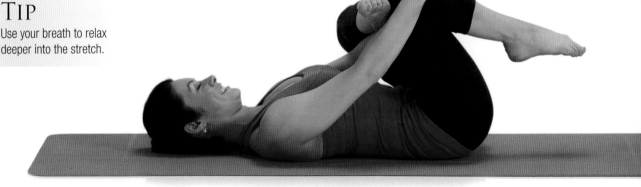

SIMPLIFY
Take one leg towards your body, drawing both the knee and the ankle closer to your chest. Repeat with the other leg.

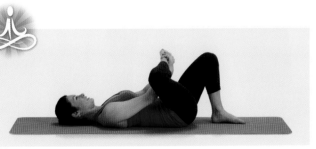

Hip Flexor Stretch

1 Kneeling on one leg, place your other foot forward with your knee directly above your ankle, avoiding a deep knee flexion.

2 Ensure both hips are aligned. Exhale and tuck your tailbone under. Inhale and hold this position.

3 Repeat the exhale and inhale 12–15 times, increasing the pelvic tilt on each exhale and sustaining the tilt on each inhale. Repeat on the other leg.

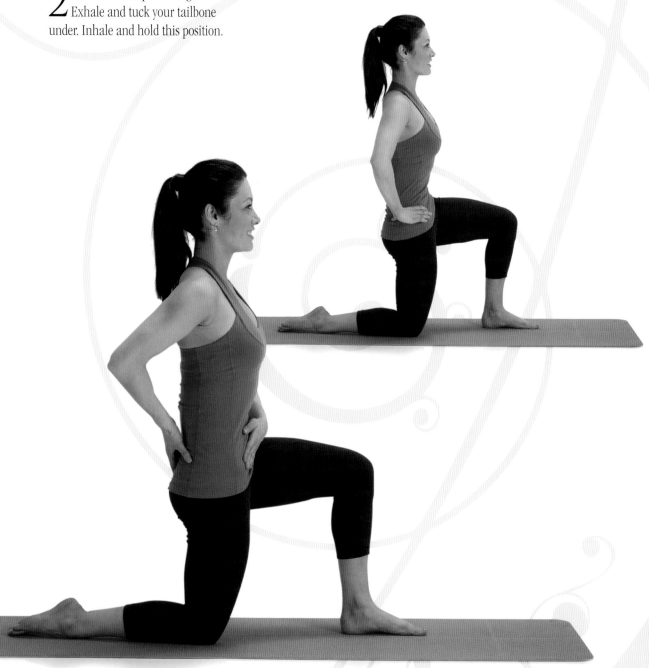

Roll Down with Calf Raise

1 Standing upright, place your feet in a 'V' position, with your heels together and your toes pointing outward.

2 Exhale and engage your stabilisers. As your organs rise internally, rise up onto your toes, simultaneously floating your arms upward.

3 Inhale, lower your heels and your arms, and prepare to roll down, flexing your cervical spine initially.

4 Exhale and flex your spine towards the floor one vertebra at a time. Inhale, hold and rest into the stretch at the bottom.

5 Exhale, engage your stabilisers, and slowly roll up to standing, restacking each vertebra with concentration and elongation.

6 Repeat 12–15 times.

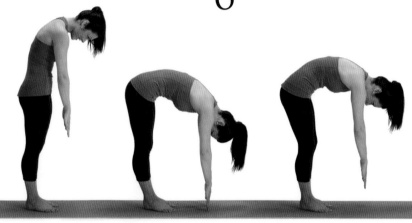

TIP
If your hamstrings and lumbar spine feel tight, ease the stretch by softly bending your knees as you roll down and hold the stretch at the bottom.

SIMPLIFY
Using a wall to lean against, position your feet your own foot-length away from the wall and allow your spine to roll on and off the wall. This modification allows for feedback on your alignment.

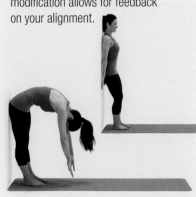

INTENSIFY
Keep your calves raised throughout the movement and try to roll down while remaining on your toes – an extremely challenging variation!

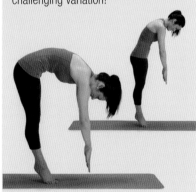

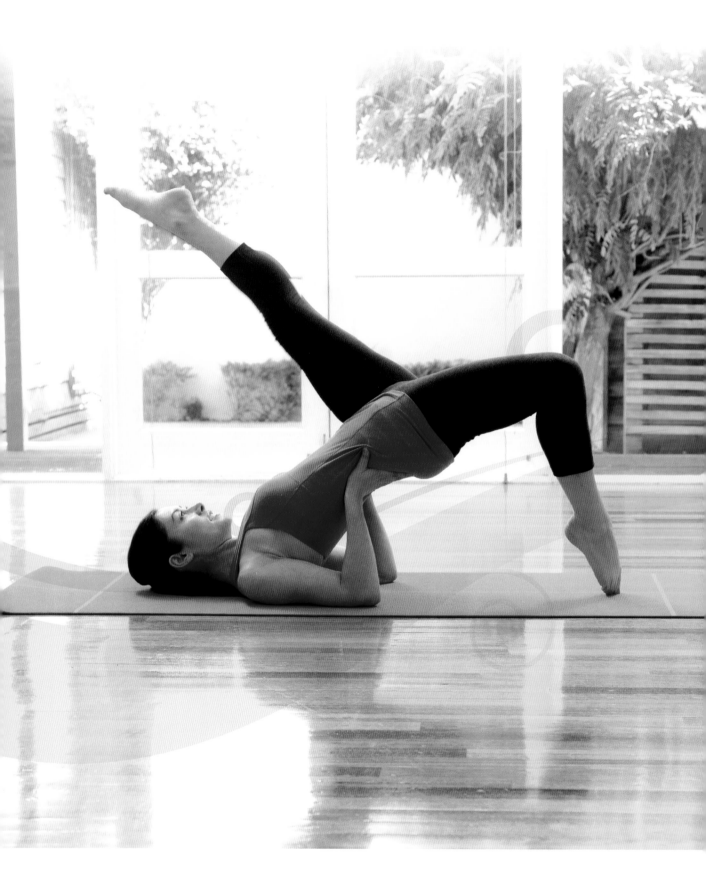

PILATES FOR WEIGHT LOSS

WORKOUTS

To assist your progress and achieve targeted results, try these specially designed programs.

BASIC CONNECTIONS

This workout outlines the best way to commence your Pilates program. Repeat this workout at least three to five times before attempting the rest of the exercises.

1. Essential Connections (all exercises)
2. Fundamentals (all exercises)
3. Gluteal Stretch
4. Hip Flexor Stretch
5. Roll Down with Calf Raise

ABDOMINAL FOCUS

This program focuses on reshaping the waist and toning the abdominals. Practise it twice a week for a balanced improvement to this area or three times a week if this is your target area.

1. Essential Connections (all exercises)
2. Fundamentals (Chest Lift, Cat Stretch, Spine Twist)
3. Roll Backs with Hamstring Stretch
4. Chest Lift with Leg Float
5. Rolling
6. Cat Stretch Push Up
7. Front Support Walks
8. Cobra

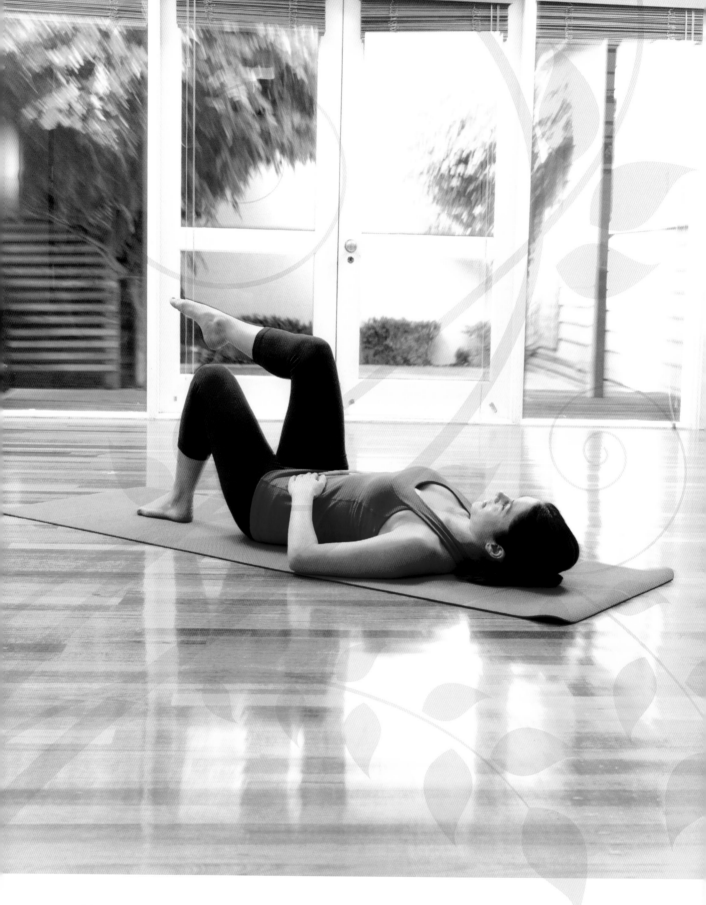

GLUTEAL & THIGH TONING

This workout targets the legs and buttocks. Practise it two to three times a week for good results, particularly if you do cardio work such as running, cycling or other exercises that lead to hip flexor tension.

1. Essential Connections (all exercises)
2. Fundamentals (Pelvic Curl, Cat Stretch, Lateral Leg Float)
3. Long Clam
4. Lateral Adductor Lift
5. Single Leg Kick
6. Side Bicycle
7. Cat Stretch Push Up
8. Swan
9. Hinge Press
10. Gluteal Stretch

UPPER BODY/POSTURAL CHALLENGE

This workout is ideal for toning the arms and upper back and is a great way to improve posture for anyone who works at a desk. Practise this twice weekly for effective results, or more often if the upper arms are your focus.

1. Essential Connections (all exercises)
2. Fundamentals (Cat Stretch, Spine Twist)
3. Prone Extension with Arm Lift
4. Cobra
5. Rolling
6. Single Leg Kick
7. Cat Stretch Push Up
8. Swan
9. Arms in Hinge
10. Front Support Walks
11. Side Support
12. Roll Down with Calf Raise

BALANCE FOCUS

This workout increases overall physical harmony while improving core stabiliser function throughout the body. Include this workout in your program once a week and increase the frequency if you cross-train for sports, dance or yoga.

1. Essential Connections (all exercises)
2. Fundamentals (Pelvic Curl, Spine Twist, Lateral Leg Float)
3. Chest Lift with Leg Float
4. Rolling
5. Long Clam
6. Lateral Adductor Lift
7. Side Bicycle
8. Swan
9. Side Support
10. Front Support Walks
11. Hinge Press with Arms in Hinge
12. Roll Down with Calf Raise

WEIGHT-LOSS PLANNER

Keep track of your progress and motivate yourself with this monthly weight-loss planner. Make a photocopy for each month. Mark any efforts made towards your Pilates practice, exercise and activities, and healthy eating on the appropriate day of the month.

	1	2	3	4	5	6	7
P							
E							
HE							
	8	9	10	11	12	13	14
P							
E							
HE							

	15	16	17	18	19	20	21
P							
E							
HE							
	22	23	24	25	26	27	28
P							
E							
HE							
	29	30	31				
P							
E							
HE							

P = Pilates
E = Exercise/Activity
HE = Healthy Eating

GLOSSARY

adductors	group of muscles running down the inner thigh from the pelvis to the knee
cardiovascular	relating to the heart and blood vessels
cervical spine	relating to the seven cervical vertebrae of the upper spine, immediately below the skull
diaphragmatic	relating to the diaphragm (the muscle wall between the abdomen and the chest)
femur	thigh bone
flexion	the action of bending a joint
gluteal	relating to the muscles of the buttocks
hamstring	tendons of the knee
hip flexors	group of muscles in the hip that control movements such as raising the leg
hip rotators	group of muscles in the hip that control movements such as rotating the thigh outwards
intercostal	relating to the muscles between the ribs
lipids	compounds such as fats and oils
lumbar fascia	the sheath that binds the muscles of the lower back together
lumbar spine	relating to the five lumbar vertebrae of the lower back
neuromuscular	relating to both the nerves and the muscles
oblique muscles	abdominal muscles used to rotate the torso
quadriceps	muscle group at the front of the thigh
rotator cuff	group of shoulder muscles responsible for shoulder rotation and stability
sacrum	triangular bone at the base of the spine and rear pelvic cavity; sits between the two pelvic bones
thoracic spine	relating to the twelve thoracic vertebrae of the middle back
thorax	chest area containing the heart and lungs
transversus abdominis	muscle running from the side to the front of the abdomen; the deepest of the major abdominal muscles

CONCLUSION

Pilates is the most efficient exercise method available for creating a toned and sleek physique. With regular practice, this exercise program will provide endless options for physical strength and personal wellbeing. Continue your healthy outlook by combining equal amounts of fun and activity with a balanced diet for optimum vitality.

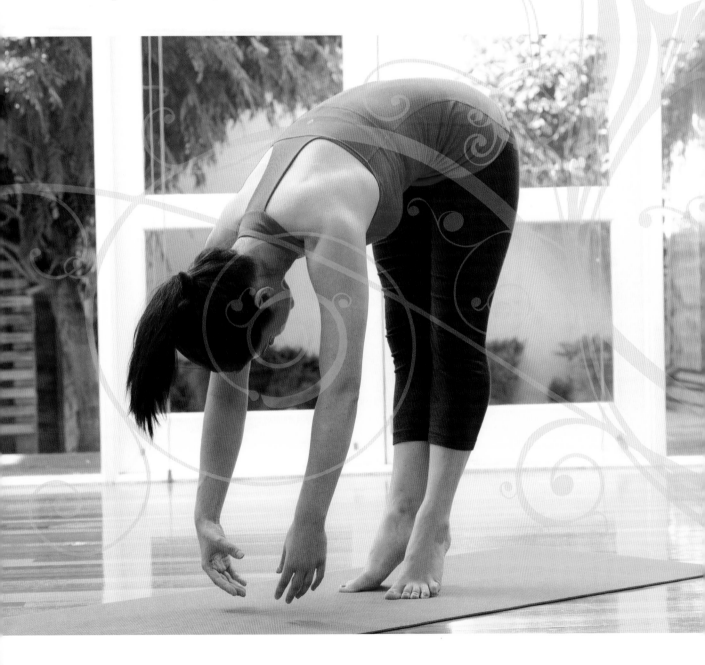

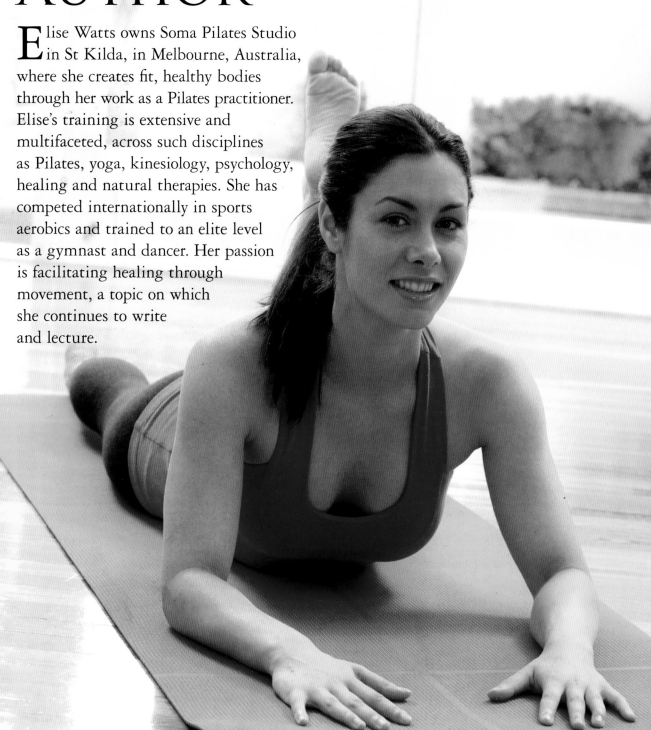

ABOUT THE AUTHOR

Elise Watts owns Soma Pilates Studio in St Kilda, in Melbourne, Australia, where she creates fit, healthy bodies through her work as a Pilates practitioner. Elise's training is extensive and multifaceted, across such disciplines as Pilates, yoga, kinesiology, psychology, healing and natural therapies. She has competed internationally in sports aerobics and trained to an elite level as a gymnast and dancer. Her passion is facilitating healing through movement, a topic on which she continues to write and lecture.

Yikes-Lice!

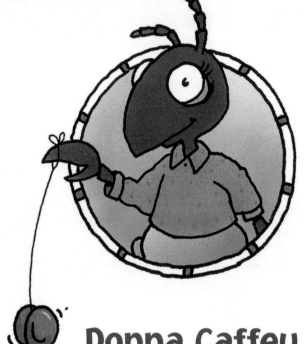

Donna Caffey

illustrations by **Patrick Girouard**

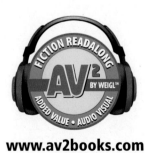

www.av2books.com

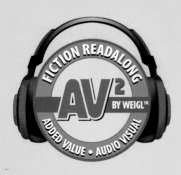

Your AV² Media Enhanced book gives you a fiction readalong online. Log on to www.av2books.com and enter the unique book code from this page to use your readalong.

AV² Readalong Navigation

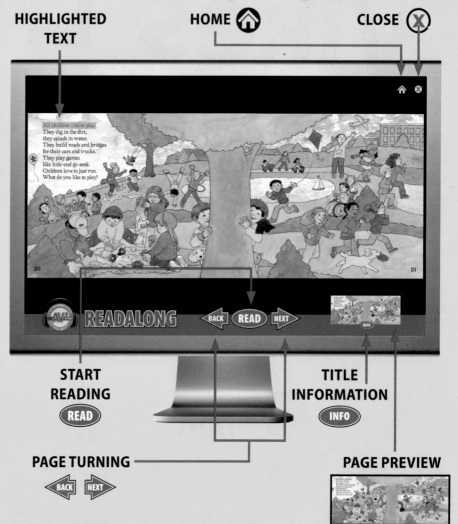

HIGHLIGHTED TEXT

HOME

CLOSE

START READING
READ

PAGE TURNING
BACK NEXT

TITLE INFORMATION
INFO

PAGE PREVIEW

Go to **www.av2books.com**, and enter this book's unique code.

BOOK CODE

S 5 0 4 2 6 7

AV² by Weigl brings you media enhanced books that support active learning.

First Published by

ALBERT WHITMAN & COMPANY
Publishing children's books since 1919

Published by AV² by Weigl
350 5ᵗʰ Avenue, 59ᵗʰ Floor New York, NY 10118
Website: www.av2books.com   www.weigl.com

Library of Congress Control Number: 2013940836

ISBN 978-1-62127-912-9 (hardcover)
ISBN 978-1-48961-503-9 (single-user eBook)
ISBN 978-1-48961-504-6 (multi-user eBook)

Printed in the United States of America in North Mankato, Minnesota
1 2 3 4 5 6 7 8 9 0   17 16 15 14 13

Text copyright ©1998 by Donna Jaye Caffey.
Illustrations copyright ©1998 by Patrick Girouard.
Published in 1998 by Albert Whitman & Company.

2 052013
WEP250413

A note to Concerned Grownups

People sometimes think that head lice are a sign of uncleanliness, but in fact anyone, no matter how clean, can get them. They are easily passed by being in close contact with someone or by sharing combs, brushes, or hats. It can be irritating and disturbing to feel head lice on your scalp, but they are not known to carry any human disease.

Young children have higher rates of head lice infestation than older children and adults. Children between the ages of three and ten are the most likely to get them. In this age group, boys and girls tend to be at equal risk. Among teenagers, girls are more often affected than boys. White children are more likely to get head lice than are African-American children.

Desperate parents have tried many household remedies, some of them dangerous and all of them unproven. Children have occasionally been seriously harmed from these home remedies, which have included commercial pesticides, kerosene, and gasoline.

Several treatments are available in pharmacies, over-the-counter, or by prescription. Some studies have suggested that lice may be gaining resistance to some of these treatments. I have been participating in a current study to determine whether available treatments are still as effective as they once were in the United States. Until research gives us new answers, the best way to deal with lice is to carefully follow the instructions given in the lice treatment packages, taking care to thoroughly remove all the lice and nits.

And remember, although head lice are a nuisance, they are not something to be feared.

Christine G. Hahn, M.D.

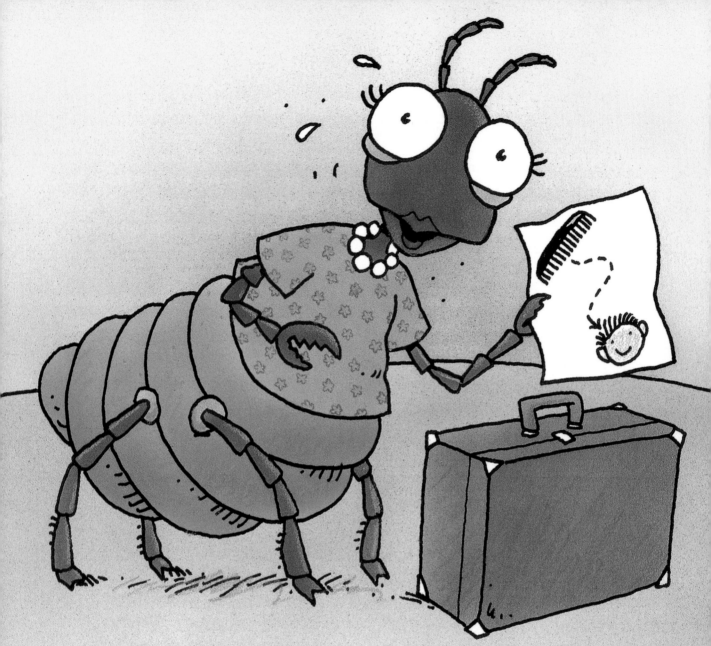

A cootie with an attitude
crept forth one day in search of food.
I'm starvin'!

The head louse, sometimes called a cootie, lives on the human head. It is a wingless insect 1/16 to 1/8 inch long, about the size of a pinhead. Head lice (the plural of louse) range in color from light brown to dark brown or black. They do not live on animals. A head louse crawls, but it does not hop, jump, or fly.

4

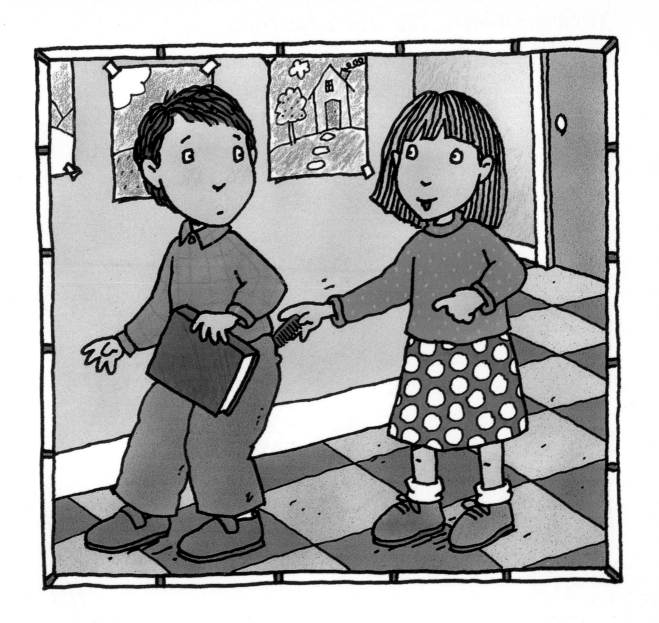

She hitched a ride on someone's comb
and went to find a great new home.
Thanks for the lift!

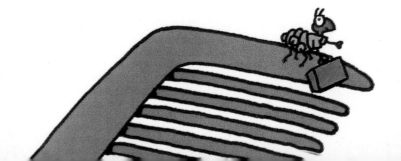

Tired and hungry, she saw some food;
a yummy meal soon changed her mood.
Mmmm!

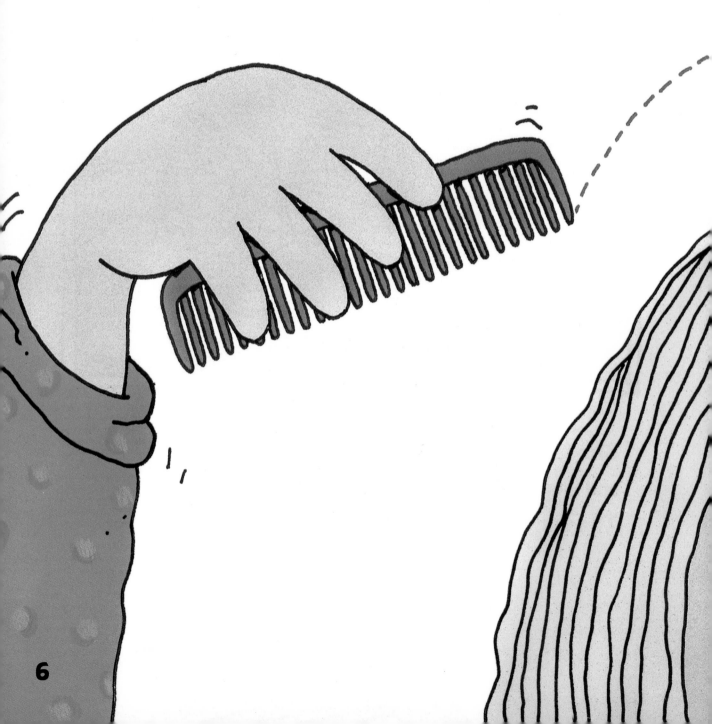

Lice are usually found nestled in the hair close to the scalp at the top of the head, behind the ears, or at the back of the neck. They have six legs, with claws used for holding onto hair.

Lice require blood from the "host," or human being they are living on, in order to survive. They use their sucking mouth parts to pierce the skin and feed. If left alone, lice will feed quickly and frequently. Without a meal, they cannot live more than one or two days.

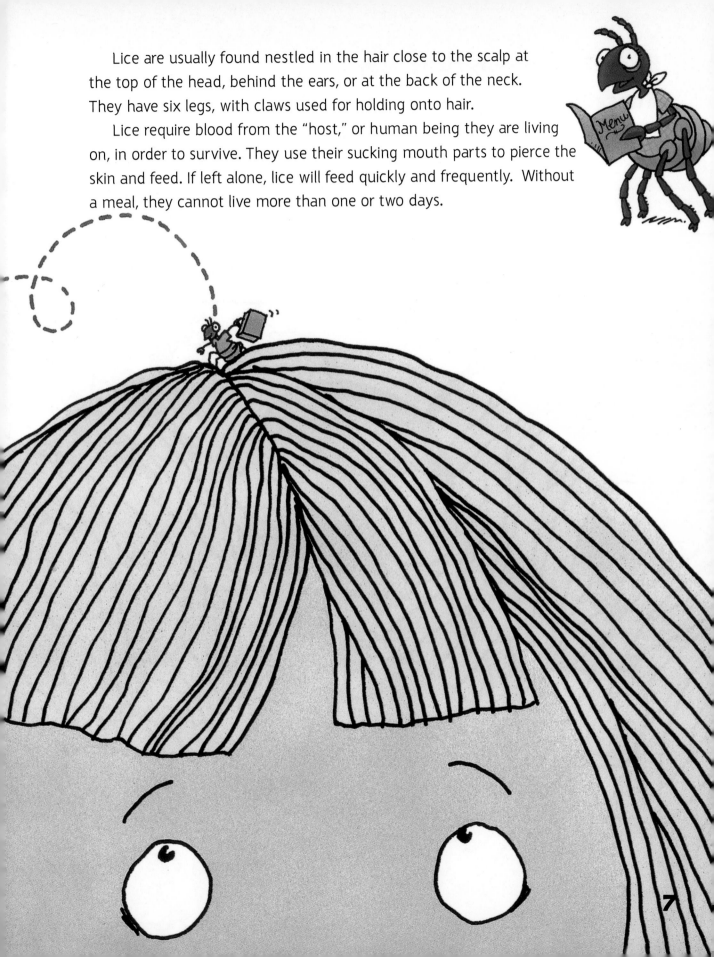

7

She raised a family right away.

Those kids played hide and seek all day.

Ready or not, here I come!

The female louse can lay 3 to 6 eggs per day—about 50 to 150 in her lifetime. The eggs, called nits, are very small (about 1/32 of an inch in length), oval-shaped, and grayish-white. The female attaches the nits to hair with a gummy substance.

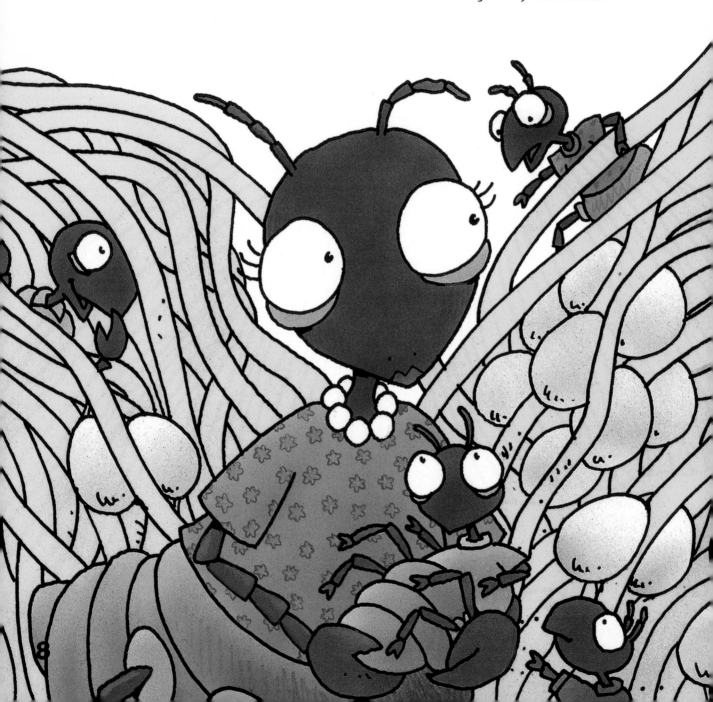

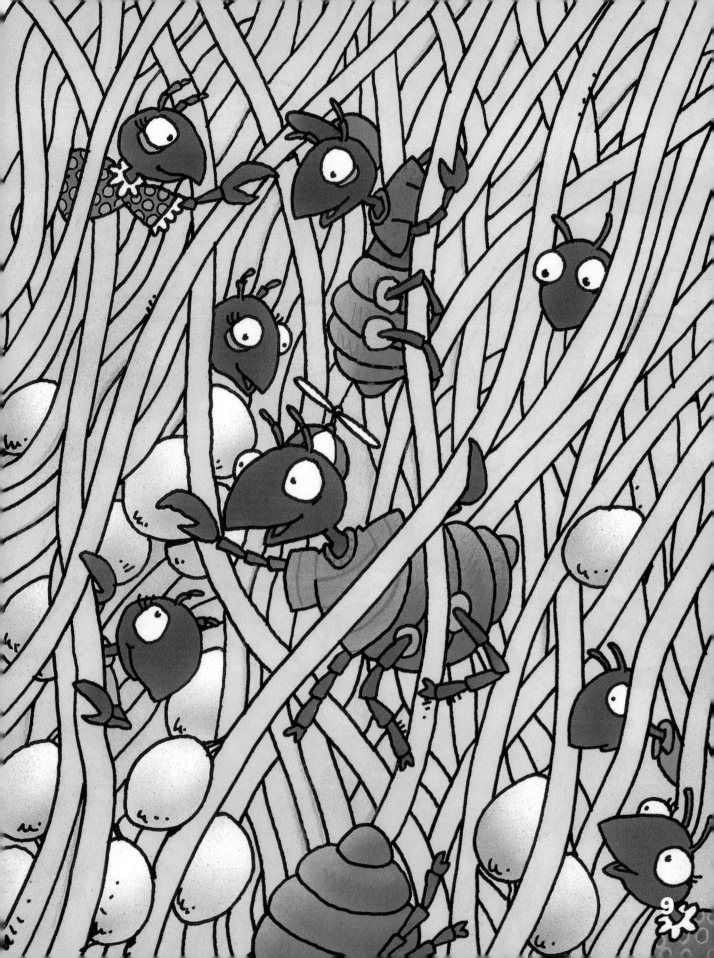

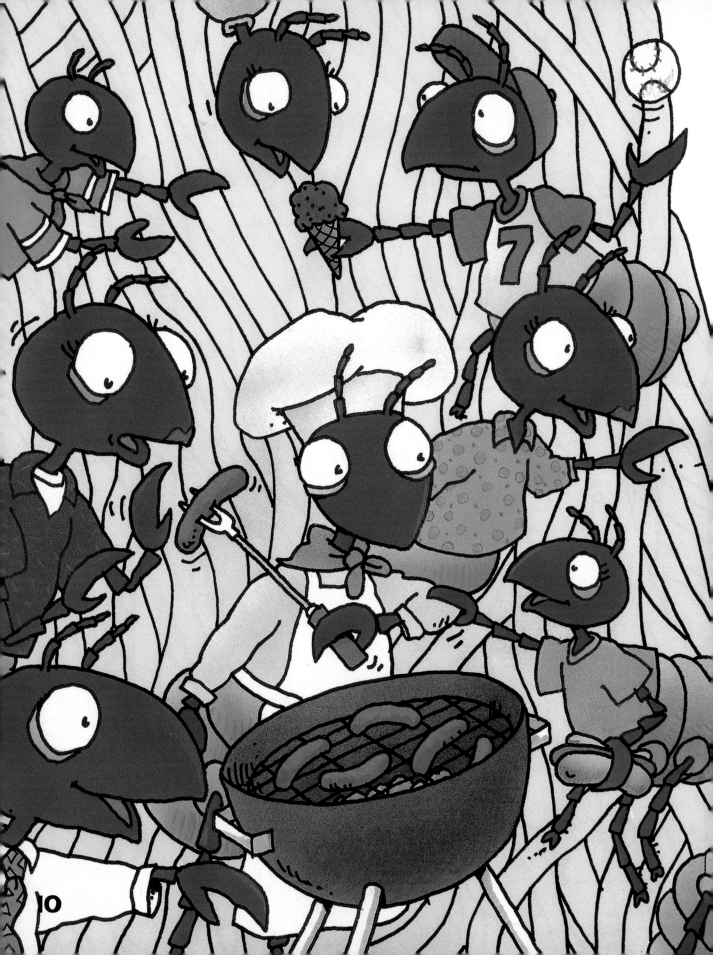

Her little ones grew up quite quick,
had tykes themselves, and stayed real thick.
A family reunion!

It takes seven to ten days for a nit to hatch and the young louse, or nymph, to emerge. Soon the nymphs mature into adults. Then the female can lay eggs of her own. Most lice live about a month, long enough to have many children and grandchildren.

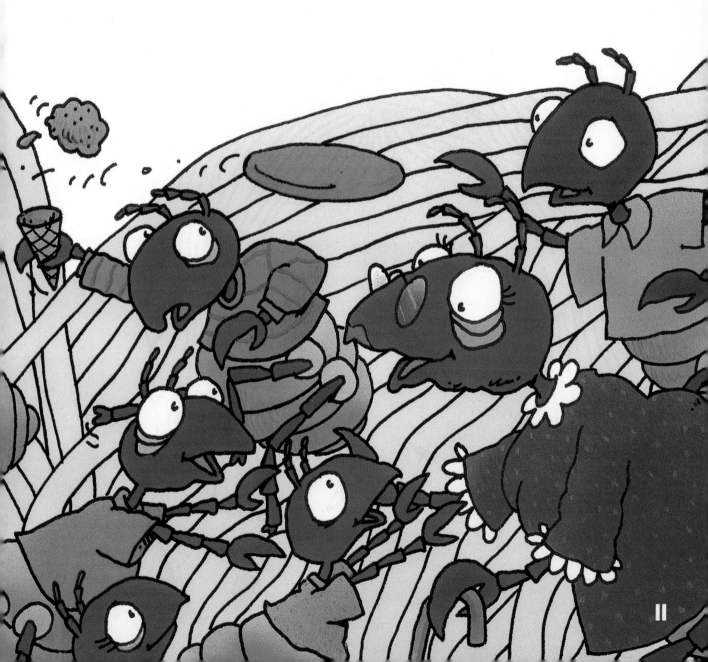

Meanwhile—

my head began to creep and crawl

with these intruders weird and small.

What was up?

If your head itches a lot, you should be checked for lice! The itching is caused by the feeding louse who punctures the skin, injects saliva, and then sucks blood. However, you can have lice and not itch.

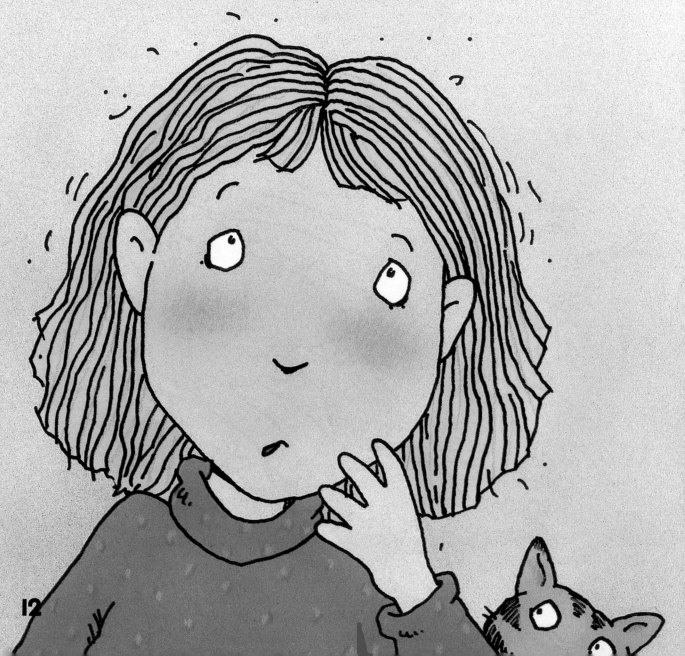

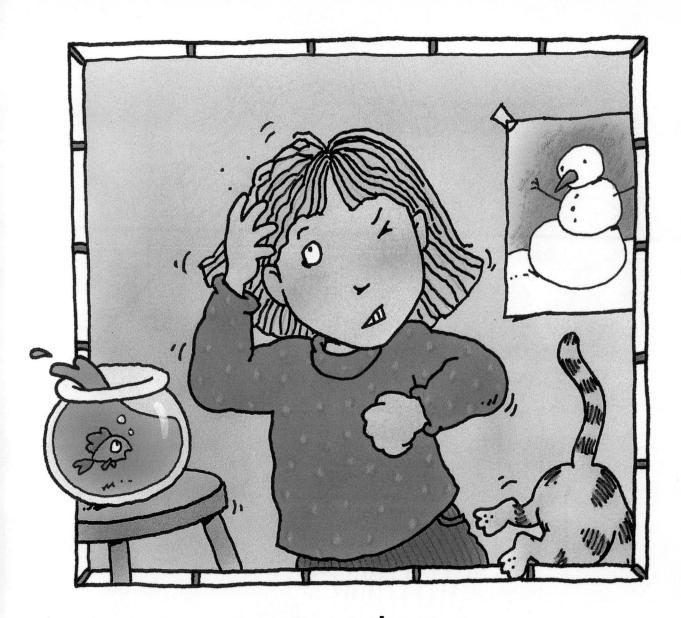

I scratched my head from neck to top.
It itched so much I couldn't stop!
Ugh!

Although they will not hurt you, head lice can be very
aggravating. They do not cause other diseases, but if
you scratch too much and break the skin, an infection
can develop.

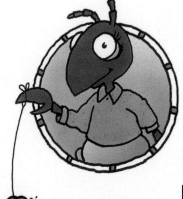

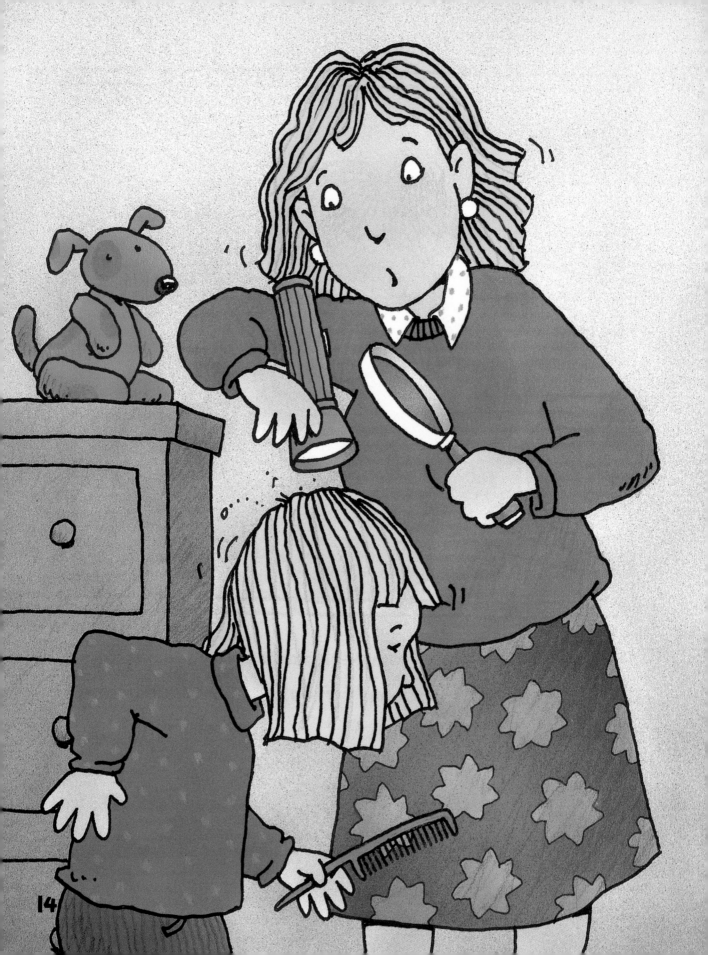

I yelled at Mom to come and look.
She grabbed a light. She glared, then shook!
Yikes!

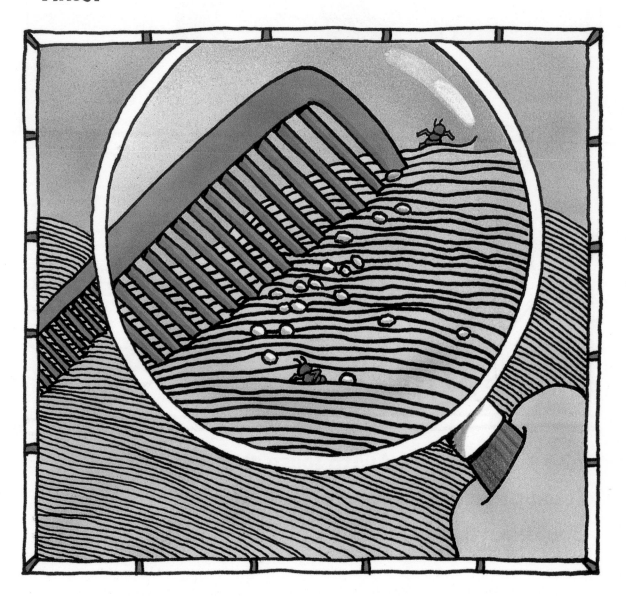

You will need help to check yourself for head lice. Lean forward under a good light. The "checker" can use a comb with a tail to part and lift the hair. He or she should begin at the back of the neck and proceed to each side, lifting the hair in small sections all over the head. Most lice and nits can be seen with the naked eye, but a magnifying glass might be helpful. (Be sure everyone's hands and all the equipment are washed after the examination.)

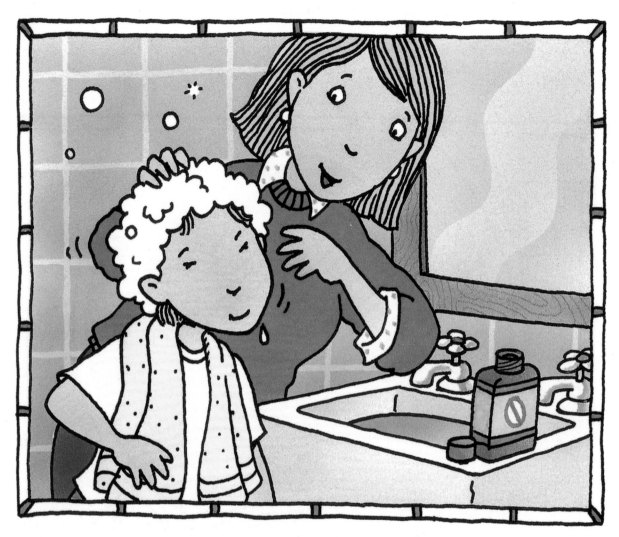

She soaped my head with louse shampoo.

It zapped those pests. I yelled, "Yahoo!"

You're outta here!

If you have lice, your hair can be washed with a louse-killing shampoo or rinse. There are several kinds you can buy. The instructions on the package should be carefully followed. If you have questions, ask your doctor. Anyone who has been in close contact with a person with lice should also be checked for lice.

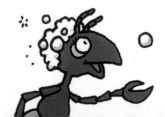

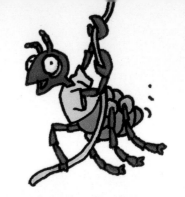

She combed my hair out over a towel; the snarls and tangles made me growl.
OUCH!

All the nits must be removed from your hair. Otherwise, they'll hatch and you'll have more lice. You'll need someone to help you get the nits out. The helper should use a nit-removal comb (these combs are often sold with lice shampoo) and work one section of hair at a time. It may be easier for someone to use his or her fingers to pull out the sticky, seedlike nits.

Combing out nits can take awhile, so be patient! It's very important to get every single one.

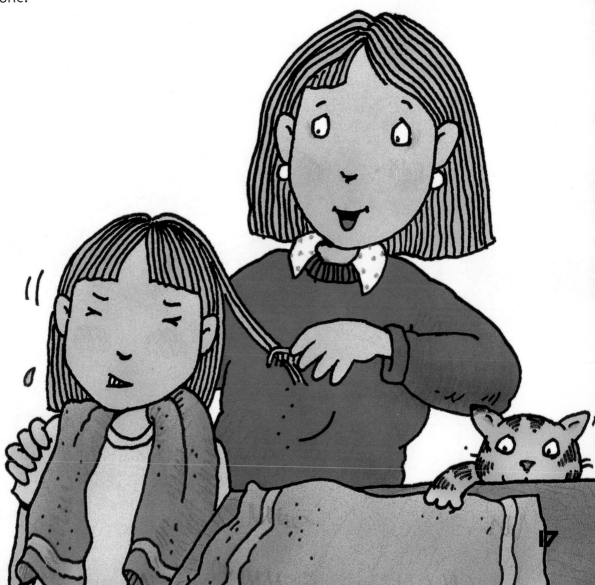

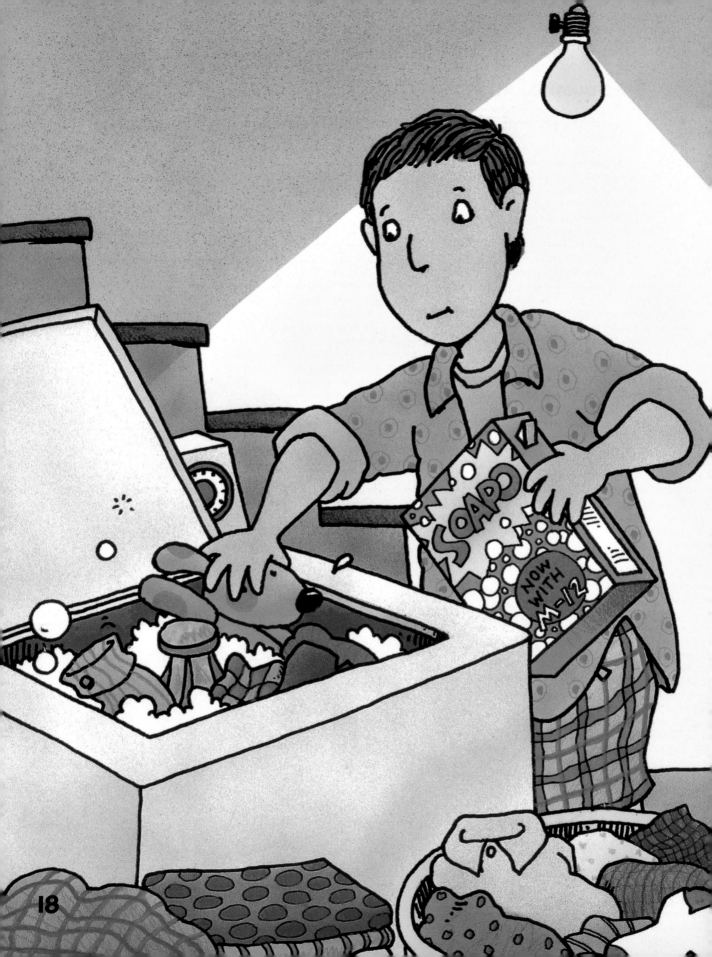

18

**Dad pitched in to start the chore
of cleaning stuff we shouldn't ignore.
Even Ole Blue!**

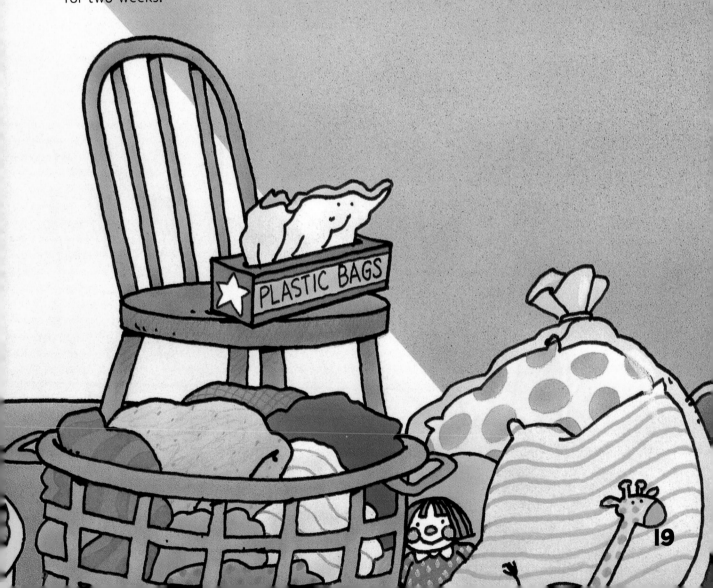

To make sure that lice are completely gone, everything that was exposed must be thoroughly cleaned. Personal items such as combs, brushes, and hair accessories must be soaked in very hot (but not boiling) water for twenty minutes. Clothing, linens, and towels should be washed with hot soapy water and completely dried in a clothes dryer using the hot cycle. Nonwashable items such as some stuffed animals, pillows, bedspreads, bike helmets, and headsets with foam earpieces, should be dry-cleaned or placed in an airtight plastic bag for two weeks.

PLASTIC BAGS

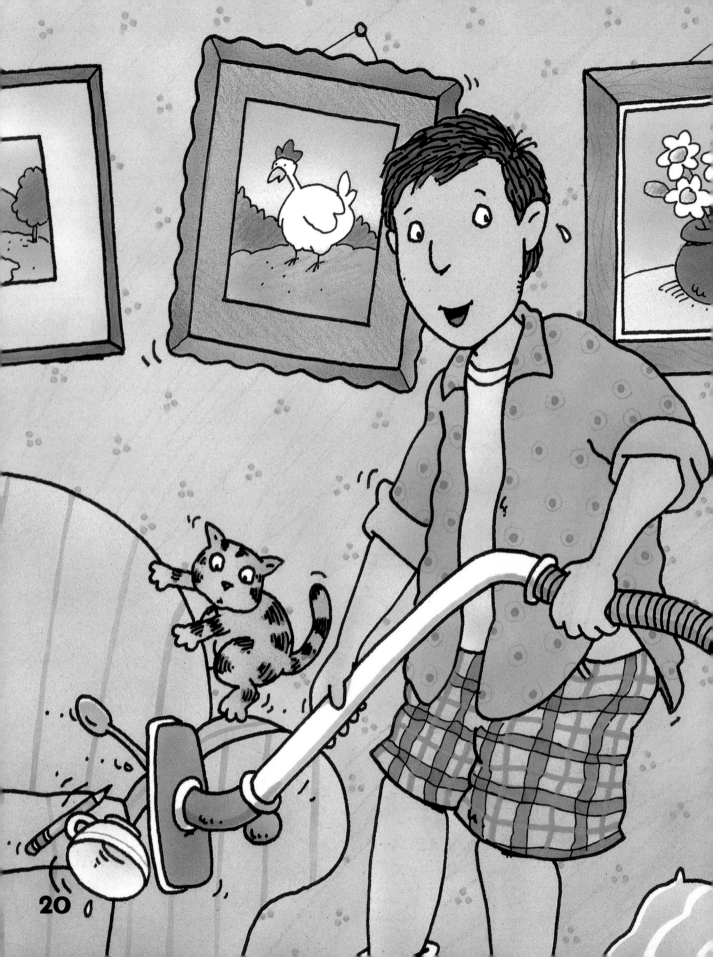

He swept the sofa, chairs, and rugs, to clean our house of all stray bugs. Whew!

Because lice can live from one to two days away from a person, sofas, chairs, mattresses, carpets, and car upholstery should be thoroughly vacuumed. Throw the vacuum bag away.

But you do not need to spray the house with insecticides. Remember that lice don't live long away from people, and you do not want to expose yourself to unnecessary chemicals.

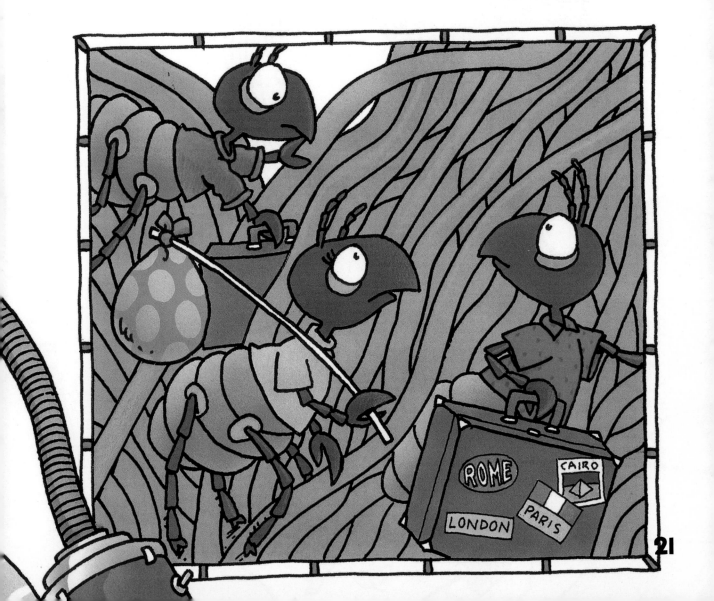

Our work complete, we had a chat.
Dad warned me not to share my hat.
No way!

Often people get lice in schools and camps or anywhere they are in close contact. It helps if you do not share your combs, brushes, hats, helmets, headsets, or clothes. If you do get lice, you should tell your teachers and friends so they can be checked. You should be checked again every day for two weeks and regularly after that.

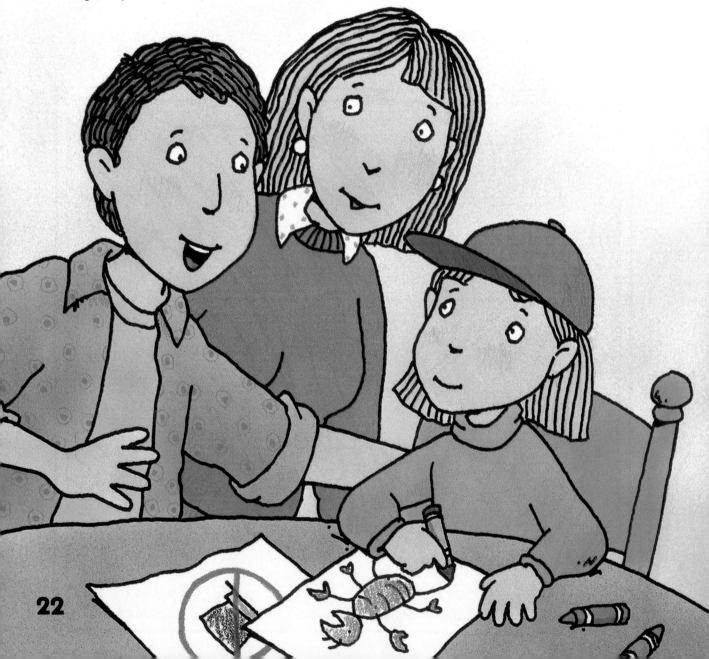

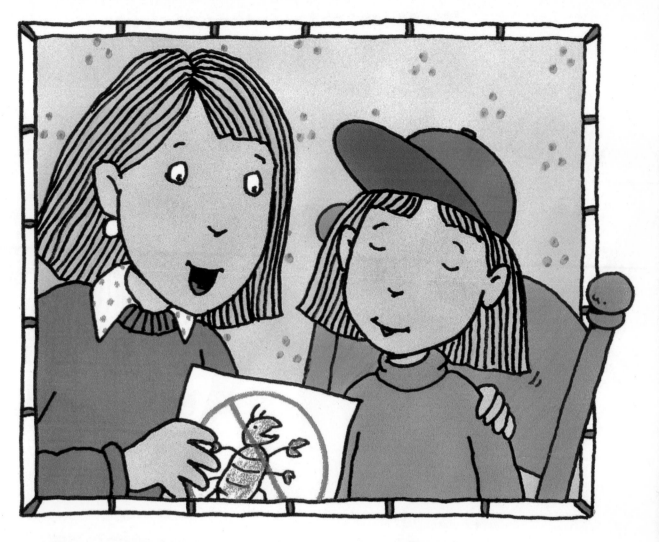

**Mom said, "You don't deserve the blame.
It's not your fault those cooties came."
That's right!**

It's not your fault if you get head lice—anyone can! According to historians, head lice have been around for nine thousand years. They have been found on people of all races all over the world, no matter where they are living or how clean they are.

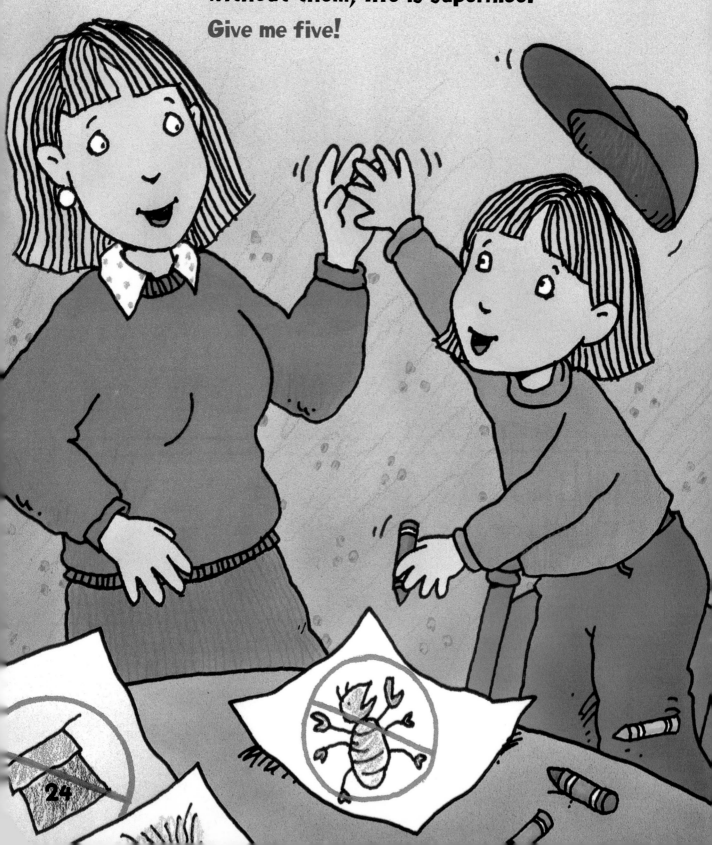

We fought and won the war on lice;
without them, life is supernice!
Give me five!

24